Bone Healing

A Wonder Herb With Bone Healing Properties

(The Complete Nutritional Guide to Reversing Bone Disease)

Joseph Bender

Published By **Phil Dawson**

Joseph Bender

All Rights Reserved

Bone Healing: A Wonder Herb With Bone Healing Properties (The Complete Nutritional Guide to Reversing Bone Disease)

ISBN   978-0-9952447-9-5

No part of this guidebook shall be reproduced in any form without permission in writing from the publisher except in the case of brief quotations embodied in critical articles or reviews.

Legal & Disclaimer

The information contained in this book is not designed to replace or take the place of any form of medicine or professional medical advice. The information in this book has been provided for educational & entertainment purposes only.

The information contained in this book has been compiled from sources deemed reliable, and it is accurate to the best of the Author's knowledge; however, the Author cannot guarantee its accuracy and validity and cannot be held liable for any errors or omissions. Changes are periodically made to this book. You must consult your doctor or get professional medical advice before using any of the suggested remedies, techniques, or information in this book.

Table Of Contents

Chapter 1: What Is Joint Pain?

Joint pain is commonplace and commonly felt in the fingers, ft, hips, knees, or backbone. Pain can be non-prevent or it would come and go. Sometimes the joint might also moreover experience tight, achy, or painful. Some sufferers file a sizzling, throbbing, or "grating" feeling. In addition, the joint may additionally additionally appear tight in the morning however loosen up and revel in higher with motion and exercising. However, an excessive amount of exercise could probably make the soreness worse. Joint ache may moreover alter the feature of the joint and may obstruct a person's capacity to perform easy actions. Severe joint ache may also damage the splendid of lifestyles. Treatment should pay interest now not honestly on ache however additionally on the impacted sports activities and functioning.

Who is extra liable to enlarge joint pain?

Joint pain has a bent to effect people who:

Have suffered beyond accidents to a joint.

Repeatedly make use of and/or abuse a muscle.

Have arthritis or one-of-a-kind continual clinical issues.

Suffer from unhappiness, tension, and stress.

Are obese.

Suffer from terrible fitness.

Age also a function in tight and painful joints. After years of utilization, and put on and strain on joints, problems may emerge in center-aged or older folks.

What reasons joint ache?

The maximum commonplace motives of continual ache in joints are:

Osteoarthritis, a not unusual kind of arthritis, arises over time due to the fact the cartilage, the protective cushion in many of the bones, wears away. The joints end up uncomfortable and inflexible. Osteoarthritis develops slowly and commonly seems all through middle existence.

Rheumatoid arthritis is a chronic situation that reasons swelling and pain inside the joints. Often the joints come to be distorted (commonly taking area within the fingers and wrists) (normally taking area within the hands and wrists).

Gout is a painful sickness wherein crystals from the body gather inside the joint, causing severe pain and swelling. This typically occurs in the big toe.

Bursitis is because of overuse. It is often present inside the hip, knee, elbow, or shoulder.

Viral infections, redness, or fever may moreover make joint mobility uncomfortable.

Injuries, at the aspect of fractured bones or sprains.

Tendinitis is an infection of the tendons or the bendy bands that link bone and muscle. It is commonly located within the elbow, heel, or shoulder and is often due to overuse.

How is joint soreness dealt with?

Although there might not be a remedy for the pain, it may be dealt with to provide the affected person comfort. Sometimes the ache may work away with the resource of taking over-the-counter treatment, or via finishing simple each day sports. In awesome instances, the ache can be indicating troubles that may handiest be remedied with prescription medicine or surgical treatment.

Simple at-home remedy options, which includes putting a heating pad or ice at the bothered region, can be counseled for short periods, a couple of instances an afternoon. Soaking in a heat tub can also bring remedy.

Exercise may moreover assist deliver returned power and function. Walking, swimming, or a few different low-impact aerobic pastime is suggested. Those who partake in immoderate wearing sports or sports activities activities sports activities may need to tone it down or increase a low-impact training plan. Gentle stretching sporting activities can also assist. Check with the scientific medical doctor earlier than beginning or continuing any workout habitual.

Weight reduction can also be advised, if required, to restrict pressure on joints.

Acetaminophen, or anti inflammatory medicinal drugs (ibuprofen), can also assist alleviate the soreness. Both of these tablets are accessible over-the-counter, notwithstanding the truth that more dosages might also additionally require a physician's prescription. Whether you have were given were given a facts of belly ulcers, renal contamination, or liver disorder, check together together together with your doctor to decide if this is the precise desire for you.

Topical treatments, along side ointments or gels that can be massaged into the skin over the troubled joint vicinity, might also moreover furthermore assist reduce pain.

Some of them may be obtained over the counter, or the medical doctor may additionally additionally write a prescription.

Dietary dietary supplements, including glucosamine, can also moreover help alleviate pain. Ask the health practitioner earlier than using any over-the-counter dietary supplements.

If the drugs or remedies do no longer alleviate the discomfort, the medical physician also can moreover prescribe:

Supportive devices, including a brace, cane, or orthotic tool within the shoe, can assist aid the joint to sell ease of movement. The clinical doctor, bodily or occupational therapist or social employee is probably able to assist with the proper choice(s) to be had.

Physical or Occupational Therapy, together with a balanced exercising habitual, may additionally step by step help lessen ache and growth flexibility.

Antidepressants can be advocated to beneficial aid enhance sleep for a affected man or woman suffering from joint pain.

Steroids, regularly given via manner of injection into the joint, provide short-time period remedy of ache and swelling.

Painkilling medicinal drugs that help alleviate pain.

Please do not forget that medicine, collectively with those available over-the-counter, influences human beings in a special way. What permits one man or woman might not art work for every other. Be nice to comply with the doctor's recommendation cautiously even as taking any drug, and notify her or him if you enjoy any lousy effects.

What may be finished to treat joint pain?

Surgery may be a opportunity if the joint pain is long-term and does not decorate with drug remedies or bodily treatment and workout. Please be cautious to talk about this with the medical doctor to ensure that the surgical operation makes experience.

There are numerous unique surgical options to be had, in conjunction with:

1. Arthroscopy: A surgical remedy wherein a physician makes or 3 tiny incisions inside the flesh above the joint and goes in the joint using an arthroscope, or a skinny, bendy, fiberoptic device, to restore cartilage or dispose of bone chips in or throughout the joint.

2. Joint substitute: If severa restoration processes do now not assist, surgical treatment can be required to replace the joint after the cartilage that cushions and protects the ends of the bones step by step wears away. This can be completed for the hip, knee, and shoulder joints. A health practitioner gets rid of sections of the affected person's bone and installs a prosthetic joint crafted from metal or plastic. This remedy has had achievement and the majority of sufferers experience prolonged-

lasting pain consolation following this kind of surgical procedure.

What signs of joint pain are grounds for state of affairs?

Symptoms of joint pain variety from mild to disabling. Without cartilage, bones rub immediately toward every extremely good because of the reality the joint moves. Symptoms can encompass:

Swelling.

Stiff or swollen joint.

Numbness.

Noisy joints, or clicking, grinding or breaking noises while shifting the joint.

Painful movement.

Difficulty bending or straightening the joint.

Loss of movement.

A pink and heated and swollen joint (This want to be evaluated rapid through a health practitioner)

When ought to I visit a scientific physician?

If pain is interfering with ordinary daily lifestyles sports activities, it's time to speak to a doctor about the trouble. It is critical to diagnose the reason of the ache fast and start treatment to alleviate pain and maintain healthful, functioning joints.

You must see a physician if:

Pain is accompanied with the resource of a fever.

There is unexplained weight loss (10 kilos or more).

Chapter 2: Mobility And Systematic Approach

You can educate your body to bend the equal way you train it to be sturdy: often and often.

So you want to emerge as cellular:

You have visions of descending right into a deep squat effectively, of turning into the person that can fold ahead proper right into a pancake posture. Or likely your ambitions are a touch tons less formidable. Maybe you actually need an awesome way to lean down and not enjoy like matters are about to explode.

Mobility is large proper now:

Mobility courses (which can be first rate from yoga sessions) are cropping up everywhere in the country. The capability to move with control appeals to human beings; so does the potential to perform incredible, acrobatic feats, maximum of which call for a alternatively excessive degree of mobility. Attaining a excessive degree of mobility needs enjoy, tough work, and an facts of the manner to be in situations. We'll check those notions beneath.

How Far Can You Flex?

The fastest approach to start having access to new tiers of movement in a joint is to isolate and circulate each joint. Isolating a joint implies deliberately moving one component without transferring others. The feasible ranges of mobility in all three dimensions is known as a joint's tiers of freedom (DOF). If you have quite a few mobility available at your joint, however don't have the power to govern the motion, you may feel together with you don't have lots electricity or lack stability.

On the other hand, in case you don't have an excessive amount of mobility handy at a joint, you have low DOFs at that unmarried joint. This need to make the joint seem like it's so stable that it's stiff. If you're that specialize in mobility, growing the DOFs at every joint with manipulate will offer you greater movement possibilities, and preferably, permit you to skip in a more coordinated fashion. Let's do not forget you're warming up your ankles before your exercise.

You execute ankle circles in your decrease back on the equal time as speakme with the individual subsequent to you. Your ankle circles are greater like knee circles due to the fact your whole lower leg is shifting in a round motion and your toes are doing bizarre furling movements. Are you in truth warming up your ankles? Not absolutely. You aren't setting apart the joint or improving your attention of strategies the joint actions. Now expect you're laying on your once more, concentrating on your foot. Can you glide your foot up and down with out moving the decrease leg? Can you hold the toes silent and feel the motion on the ankle? Now, are you able to drift the foot inside and outside, despite the truth that with out using the feet or the lower leg? Now try connecting the dots, generating an ankle circle. Keep the whole thing else calm, keeping apart the movement at the ankle.

This may be one-of-a-type from the ankle circle noted above. Maximizing managed DOFs allows you to self-prepare better whilst peculiar matters rise up, like when you have to scale a fence to gain the route on the alternative facet. Or, for the plenty tons much less courageous readers, at the same time as there may be an sick-positioned puddle and you don't want to get your new footwear moist). If your joints carry out nicely by myself, they may paintings properly collectively. Isolated joint warm temperature-americaalso will let you become aware of in which your sticky places are. They enchantment to hobby to disparities between the 2 facets of the body. When performed constantly, isolated joint warmness-u.S. Of americalead to a complex range of motion and better tiers of joint control.

Stretching and Your Nervous System

There are branches of the demanding gadget: the sympathetic and the parasympathetic. These branches art work collectively to installation a balance among being aware and prepared to tackle the area, and sitting at the couch, browsing the net. When there can be some thing possibly dangerous that might motive harm to the organism (you), the sympathetic hectic system turns matters up and muscular tissues end up stiff. Imagine someone sneaking up at the back of you and putting his fingers difficult on your returned.

How may additionally need to you reply? I bet genuinely the belief of that makes your muscle groups anxious. Your sympathetic hectic system may be on high alert to evaluate in case you need to fight or run. Now take into account you're sitting in a hot bathtub after a ninety-minute rub down. How may also your muscle groups experience? Probably pretty calm. With no instantaneous chance lurking, your parasympathetic traumatic device might be telling you it's k to stay calm and restful.

If I informed you to stand up and speak to your toes, would it not be less hard after you've got been taken aback, or after you bought out of the current bathtub?

For a number of us, the mere notion of leaning ahead to the touch our feet triggers an inner groan as we assume the pain. We have a propensity to live in a more compassionate state of affairs. We are constantly walking; sitting table positive is uncomfortable. We may also need to should pressure in excessive net website site visitors for paintings, or have a mission that feeds into this mind-set of continuously being "on." We pick physical video video games which is probably high-intensity and war with slowing subjects down.

When we stay around in a stretch for a extended quantity of time, not like our bendier colleagues, subjects don't sincerely revel in snug. For most humans, after they enter right into a stretch, the primary aspect that occurs is the nerve-racking system (preferably) starts offevolved to lighten up and say, "this posture can be very well. Nothing horrible goes on, so I can continue to be here for a quick while." For people like me, the involved device starts offevolved sending alarm bells, making rest hard. Instead, we're left with the overwhelming urge to fidget, along element cramping in weird places as we attempt to "soften into the stretch."

There are processes to mitigate the incapacity to lighten up via stretching, through props, and satisfactory going to the vicinity wherein you experience snug, no longer past. This lets in your concerned gadget to find out a medium floor, where the stiffness may also soften up a bit bit. Research implies sports activities along with restorative yoga with useful resource reduce sympathetic worried tool interest; one of the feasible aspect effects is probably superior flexibility.

I train yoga semi-frequently to US Navy officers. The majority fall into the "stiffer" agency, and I actually have discovered that maximizing their experience is to move mindfully, with the breath, into a feature, stay there for three or 4 breaths, then glide on. Staying in postures longer lowers their calming impact, and consequences in face contortions that aren't indicative of mindfulness.

Strength and Stretching

Maybe one of the motives you could't get into a particular stretch has less to do with the muscle groups being wound tight, and extra to do with a lack of energy. Muscles are most powerful on the equal time because the joint is flexed in its mid-range. 6 Unless you guide the muscle companies close to the save you range, they gained't be capable of actively hold the placement.

Try this: capture a dowel. Hold onto it at the back of your decrease lower returned, at the facet of your palms going via outwards. Exhale, and allow your ribs drop down. Keep the ribs on this feature as you start to actively pull your fingers away from every unique.

Your arms will start to straighten. Keep this motion of the hands pulling an extended way from every distinctive as you growth the dowel away from the body. Don't permit the ribs to shift function, and preserve the wrists right now, now not bending in or out. Make sure your shoulders don't roll ahead- bear in mind, you're pulling the palms away from each special. Relax, and allow the hands decrease backpedal. Do this ten times.

What are you experiencing?

I am going to assume you feel your triceps. Probably pretty masses. This role additionally stretches the biceps, but the feeling of the triceps artwork likely overpowers any sensation of "stretch." You are strengthening your triceps thru transferring in an out of an end-variety position. In this example, the give up range is the location wherein the muscle is the shortest (the triceps settlement to extend the arm. If the arm is in no manner really straightened, the triceps gained't ever be contracting at the shortest a part of the muscle). You also can attempt bending your proper knee at the back of you, as even though you were doing a quad stretch. But don't take hold of your foot, absolutely use muscular attempt to keep it there. The hamstrings flex the knee, however we don't regularly allow the knee really bend without giving it a piece of assist with our hand; as a cease end result, we in no way clearly artwork the hamstring in its shortest sort of movement.

Working the eccentric element of a motion is some other technique to using energy throughout a muscle's variety of motion:

The eccentric trouble of a motion comes whilst you oppose gravity.

For example, whilst you execute a body weight squat, slow down the descent, allowing the reducing phase takes instances as prolonged because it takes to climb up. The art work seems like it grows. This is similar to what takes area while you pass direction jogging for the number one time in a while.

Unless you're superhuman, your quads will revel in sore. This isn't from on foot up steep hills, however from strolling down the ones steep hills.

Your quadriceps are resisting gravity with every step so you don't come to be to your face. In every instances, you're controlling a fall. Emphasizing the eccentric part of the movement is a manner to gain control inside the course of the kind of movement available to you at the joint. It coincides with will growth each in power and flexibility, and can be an effective way to increase mobility without really "stretching."

Another manner to work on strength and enhance flexibility at the equal time is to carry out isometric contractions.

You revel in a temporary growth in strength and improvements in type of motion directly following a strong isometric motion. Nine That sounds great complicated, so permit's comply with this to an real exercise. Let's say you need to work in your hamstring power and get greater flexible. Lie down to your again close to a doorway. Place your proper leg within the doorway, at a function wherein you begin to revel in a stretch.

The left leg can either be lengthy or bent. Exhale, permit your ribs melt down, and ensure you enjoy the mid lower back in competition to the ground (we're maintaining apart the hamstring, not the pelvis or low again). Press your proper heel firmly into the entrance for 20-30 seconds. You need to experience art work in your proper hamstring. Now, raise the right heel a long manner from the wall. This need to appear pretty resultseasily. You mysteriously "extended" your variety of motion.

The Stretching Part of Stretching

I stated earlier that placing out in a feature we may want to the nervous device comprehend the area is ok. I am going to cope with this from a obviously stiff individual's detail of view. I will talk about the bendy individual in a later put up. When I started out working in the direction of yoga thirteen years ago, the feeling of stretching have become distinctly uncomfortable. Two matters have helped me drastically over the years:

1. Focus on which joints are concerned in the motion, and isolate those joints:

For instance, once I carry out a pancake stretch, I do not sense my hamstrings or my calves. I sense my abs. A lot. This is because of the fact I reputation on flexing on the hip whilst maintaining my legs sturdy. A pancake stretch is certainly a seated hip flexion with the legs wide. Once I am settled into the placement, I breathe, inhaling for a don't forget of 4 and exhaling for a matter of six, for 30-60 seconds. Breathing soothes the fearful device and overcomes the a part of your thoughts that yells, "no! I don't want to be right here!"

2. Get proper right into a feature near the point of stretch and do a little aspect there:

If you're operating on hip extension (herbal hip extension, now not lumbar extension), get right into a tall half of of-kneeling position at the facet of your proper leg decrease returned. See if you could set yourself up so you revel in robust with a experience of the begin of a stretch to your proper hip. As you exhale, boom your arm overhead. Inhale, and lower the arm down. Perform 6-8 repetitions and transfer aspects.

Stretching Might Be Long-Lasting

For instance, in advance than I squat, I dynamically and statically stretch my calves to decorate my ankle dorsiflexion. I then use that variety of motion when I squat. Over time, this has precipitated masses much less of a stretch sensation in my calves. They are becoming much less tight, in part because of repeated exposure to the stretch, and in part because I certainly have reinforced the muscle groups that assist my ankle thru way of the usage of the variety of movement.

The Systematic Mobility Program:

The capacity to move inner and out of positions is based on an interplay among your aggravating system and your frame shape. Like one in all a kind sides of training, mobility education want to be carried out in a scientific, innovative manner. If your motive is to growth the form of movement in a selected place, ask your self what you propose on the usage of the movement to do. Program your mobility paintings to enhance that interest.

Below is an example of the manner you may software a 4-week mobility skills set into your exercising. The flexibility talent is the prolonged take a seat down posture, yet the principles is probably completed to something. For all the mobility schooling, breathe in through your nose and out via each your nostril or mouth. Let the exhale be longer than the inhale. Go slowly, and discover the natural rhythm of the breath.

Weeks 1 and three

Day 1 (do honestly on week 1)

Perform your ordinary exercise. At the surrender of your exercising, come into an prolonged sitting function and take a picture (or have someone take a image) This will function a baseline.

Day 2

Warm Up: Add fame right away leg increases, keeping apart the movement on the hip joint, and ankle circles. Be wonderful to move slowly and flow into at the hip and ankle, respectively. Breathe for the duration of the movement, the usage of the exhale to elevate the leg at some stage in reputation hip flexion. Perform five on each side.

Cool Down: Lie to your lower back collectively together with your legs immediately up in opposition to a wall. Make positive you are some distance sufficient away that your pelvis doesn't roll whilst you area your leg on the wall. Exhale, press the heels into the wall; inhale, loosen up. Perform 10. On the final one, hold your legs up the wall and rest for 30-60 seconds.

Day three

Warm Up: Lie for your returned at the side of your knees bent. As you exhale, pick out up your right foot and location your hands behind your proper thigh. Your returned need to enjoy prolonged, and your ribs have to be comfortable. Make extraordinary your hips haven't shifted and your pelvis remains degree. Begin shifting in reality on the proper ankle. You would possibly probable flex and attain the heel, or skip the foot internal and out. Take approximately 60 seconds to find out motion on the ankle joint. Switch factors.

After you have finished acting the motion at the ankle, exhale and choose your proper foot up over again, taking your arms behind your right thigh. On your subsequent breath, growth the right knee, extending your right heel in the direction of the ceiling. Inhale, and lighten up it. There need to be no motion on the hip joint. Perform 10 sluggish repetitions and switch elements.

Cool Down: Sit on a few element decrease than your knees, however excessive enough that your pelvis doesn't roll backward. Your knees might be bent and your feet flat at the floor. Staying focused in your pelvis, exhale, and slide your heels earlier so your legs begin to get lengthy inside the the front of you. Make nice your feet aspect in the direction of the ceiling and your feet are close to parallel with each different. Inhale, slide lower back to starting role. Perform 10. Hold straight away to the final one collectively along with your legs extended for 30-60 seconds.

Day 4

Repeat day 2

Day 5

Repeat day 3

Weeks 2 and 4

Day 1

Warm Up: Stand on a step so the step helps the balls of your toes, your heels are off the step, your foot is flat, and you've were given some thing to hold at once to (I use the cable device). Get the feel that the load is even all through the balls of your toes and your feet are close to parallel. As you exhale, keeping the load evenly in the course of the balls of the feet, permit the heels decrease down beneath the aircraft of the step. Inhale, move returned to the start characteristic. Perform 10. Sit down on a bench together at the side of your feet flat, your hips rectangular, and your pelvis stage. As you exhale, achieve your right heel out. Your toes will factor closer to the ceiling. Once the leg is at once, see if you can enhance the straight away right leg off the floor without changing the location of your pelvis or rotating your hips far from the rectangular. Inhale, lower down and move again to the center. Perform 10 and transfer elements.

Chapter 3: The Best Therapy For Bone Fracture

A fracture is a fractured bone. Doctors will lease numerous processes to deal with bone fractures primarily based mostly on their vicinity, nature, and severity. Fractures can be fashionable or partial. Some want surgical remedy or steel plates, at the same time as others may surely need a brace. Everyone who has a damaged bone gets higher in each other way. The recovery technique will rely on the type and diploma of the damage, the stability of fracture fixation, and organic strategies, therefore a healthy restoration method is crucial.

In this newsletter, we take a look at how surgeons address bone fractures, the technological information in the once more of the three essential stages of bone restoration, and home remedies to hurry up bone healing.

Why need to you have got a bone fracture repaired?

If a person with a broken bone does no longer acquire care from a physician, there can be a capability that the bone can also mend in an uncommon function. One of the targets of treatment is to repair the natural anatomy consequently a systematic doctor will modify and reset every phase of the bone into its right anatomic vicinity.

People can also have bone fractures with numerous tiers of severity, and irrespective of the fact that some may be trivial, others can bring about principal effects. No rely how severe a bone fracture is, a person should constantly go to their doctor for treatment to save you destiny effects, together with odd recovery, lack of function, or bone deficiencies. Other outcomes of incorrectly dealt with bone fractures encompass:

The introduction of a blood clot in neighboring blood vessels.

Infection from the damage.

Damage to the pores and pores and skin, tissues, or muscle groups across the fracture.

Swelling of a close-by joint because of bleeding into the joint location.

If someone breaks a extended bone, inclusive of the thigh bone (femur), they may come across a critical impact termed a fats embolism. Here, fat globules are discharged into the circulate and deposited in the lung capillaries, ensuing in respiratory pain. If left untreated, it can be deadly.

Ways to treatment a fractured bone:

Depending on the kind and region of the damaged bone, a physician may also propose the subsequent treatments:

Traditional solid

After relocating the bone, surgeons will regularly immobilize the shattered bone with a plaster or fiberglass forged. A stable will allow the bone to get better in the proper area. Doctors commonly use casts to restore fractures within the leg, foot, arm, and wrist bones.

Functional forged or brace

A useful stable or brace varies from common solid immobilization in that it lets in confined and controlled mobility of surrounding joints. Usually, surgeons area an preliminary strong on the limb with the fractured bone and cast off it after a while. Then, the scientific health practitioner will region the limb in a practical brace, which permits its early movement and mobility.

Open cut price

When someone suffers a giant bone fracture, surgeons may also want to behavior surgery to restoration the spoil. In an open reduce rate method, surgeons find and rearrange the bone with the useful aid of hand. People also can additionally want open cut rate within the event that they have got complex fractures or fractures which are beside the aspect for treatment with a strong.

There are sorts of open cut price:

Open discount with internal fixation

This remedy consists of connecting unique screws or steel plates to the outdoors floor of the bone. The medical expert also can additionally additionally positioned metal rods inside the center of the bone to preserve the bone fragments collectively.

Open bargain with outside fixation

This treatment consists of attaching an outdoor tool to the stricken limb following surgical operation. The fitness care expert installs steel pins or screws above and under the fracture internet site to resource and immobilize the bone even as it heals.

Three ranges of bone recovery:

When someone fractures a bone, they generally go through three levels of healing:

1. The inflammatory segment.

The inflammatory section, every so often termed fracture hematoma improvement, is the initial level of restoration that takes vicinity fast after the damage. According to at least one studies, extra or lots less forty eight hours after the harm, blood vessels broken through the fracture leak blood. This blood begins offevolved to coagulate and produces a fracture hematoma. Because of the disturbance of blood deliver to the bone, some bone cells close to the fracture perish. This inflammatory level finishes spherical one week following the fracture.

2. The mending phase.

The mending or reparative section begins at some point of the primary few days following the bone fracture and lasts for round 2 - three weeks. During this era, the frame builds cartilage and tissue in and throughout the fracture net website on line. The tissue creates a smooth collar on the shattered ends of the bones, and the tissue grows till the 2 ends meet. These growths are referred to as calluses, and their function is to useful resource the fracture. Over the subsequent weeks, a bony callus made from spongy bone known as trabecular bone will replace the tissue callus.

3. Bone remodeling.

The remodeling phase is the closing step in fracture recovery. At this degree, robust bone replaces spongy bone, completing the recovery technique. Sometimes, the outer ground of the bone remains barely swollen for some time, which ought to treatment on its private.

Healing time for fractured bones:

Depending at the severity of the fracture and the way nicely someone follows their medical doctor's recommendations, bones can take amongst weeks to numerous months to heal. According to the several sanatorium reviews, the not unusual bone recuperation time is amongst 6-8 weeks, despite the truth that it could variety relying on the type and location of the harm. People regularly give up experiencing ache prolonged in advance than the fractured bone has healed and the leg is appropriate for normal exercising.

Home techniques to rush up repair:

The outstanding approach to assist bone fracture mending is to relaxation and reduce using the limb. Other techniques someone may also hire to lessen recovery time and accelerate bone healing include the following:

Take protein dietary nutritional dietary supplements

As a big part of a bone consists of protein, taking protein supplements can assist the bone to rebuild and heal itself. People with a protein deficiency can also growth a spongy callus throughout the fracture in desire to a corporation callus.

Take antioxidants

Antioxidants put off loose radicals which are created via tissue damage. Because bone fractures comprise tissue damage, the use of antioxidant supplements may also additionally resource with bone repair. People might also additionally get antioxidants in dietary supplements that include nutrients E and C, lycopene, and alpha-lipoic acid.

Take mineral dietary supplements

Bone is often composed of minerals, which encompass calcium, silicon, magnesium, phosphorus, and zinc. People might also discover that their bone heals faster inside the occasion that they increase their consumption of those minerals. These nutritional supplements might also additionally boost up callus formation, increase the manufacturing of bone protein, and accelerate the bone recovery device.

The high-quality technique to help bone fracture mending is to rest and restrict using the limb. Other strategies a person would possibly rent to decrease recuperation time and speed up bone healing encompass the subsequent:

Take diet supplements

Vitamins also are important for bone rebuilding as they promote most of the mobile techniques and reactions that rise up in bone. Vitamins C, D, and K play vital roles inside the fracture restoration machine. Vitamin B is essential for strength production.

Take herbal nutritional dietary supplements

People also can use herbal dietary supplements to hurry fracture recovery. Some human beings say that Symphytum (comfrey), arnica, and horsetail grass are probably beneficial herbs. However, typically use herbs with caution, as massive portions of those herbs can be toxic.

Exercise

Always speak to a scientific scientific doctor earlier than using exercise as a manner to rush up bone recuperation, because it will handiest be appropriate at superb stages of the healing machine. However, if completed under a medical doctor's supervision, exercise can beautify blood waft to the injured net website online, assist to rebuild muscle spherical it, and accelerate bone fracture recovery. Furthermore, some human beings also can regain limb characteristic thru exercise.

Avoid smoking

People who smoke may additionally moreover go through delayed bone repair. Sometimes, this could bring about a scenario wherein the bone does not heal and develops a non-union fracture or takes longer to heal.

Outlook

When a bone fractures, the first aspect a health practitioner will do is ready it lower decrease lower back to its specific function. They can use a whole lot of treatments to benefit this, which may additionally moreover or might not encompass surgical treatment. The volume of someone's harm and their compliance with the clinical doctor's recommendations will determine how nicely and the way quick the fracture heals. After surgical treatment or having a brace or cast eliminated, many humans will find that they have got constrained mobility for a while. Many human beings may even lose muscle inside the injured limb during recuperation, however with specific sports activities sports, they're able to frequently regain muscle electricity and versatility in the vicinity.

Falls and injuries:

Diseases and continual situations. Sports accidents. Bone fractures can show as tons as everyone at any time. But with superior remedies, and through making some life-style and nutritional changes, there are numerous ways to boost up the restoration of a bone fracture.

Chapter 4: How Your Back And Neck Operate And Why They Pain So Much

THE CULPRIT: BAD POSTURE

By a long way the most extensive purpose of decrease lower back pain and neck discomfort is bad posture.

Therefore, back pain typically accompanies the ones moves:

Sitting for an prolonged period.

Bending for an prolonged period or over and all over again typically at paintings.

Lifting massive gadgets.

Standing.

Lying down in a posture of strain.

Similarly, neck ache usually accompanies mistaken posture in responsibilities collectively with the ones:

Sitting for a long time.

Working in a strained posture (such as the workplace employee who frequently holds a telephone in place a number of the head and shoulder, or the tractor operator who frequently turns his head to take a look at the lower back of him).

Lying down or sound asleep with the pinnacle in an uncomfortable posture.

This book will assist you hold extremely good posture and allow you to do away with the pain and stiffness that arise from incorrect posture.

THE LORDOSIS

Before you start the physical video video games, you need to recognize what wrong posture is. And to reap this, you need to apprehend the definition of the term lordosis. This phrase may also moreover sound like an contamination or an dangerous situation, but in fact, it is a natural thing of the lumbar backbone in all human beings.

Lordosis is an inward bend of the backbone. The inward bend within the lower decrease lower back is called the lumbar lordosis (Fig. 2.1).

This lordosis is located inside the small of the lower back, barely above the waistline. Some human beings are attempting to find recommendation from it as the "hole" of inside the decrease lower lower returned. The lesser inward bend of the neck is referred to as the cervical lordosis. When a person stands erect, lordosis routinely arises. Still, the degree of the lordosis varies from character to individual and from hobby to interest.

Lumbar lordosis (Fig. 2.1).

Maintenance of lumbar lordosis isn't genuinely useful in the employer to make the once more healthful and pain-unfastened: it's far crucial. Nevertheless, irrespective of the reality that the lordosis is everyday and no matter its significance, it isn't always constantly located in absolutely everyone. In reality, practically everyone loses the lordosis after precise sports, like as leaning over and touching one's toes.

The lordosis is misplaced as quickly as the decrease another time is "rounded," as typically takes area even as people sit down or when they lean beforehand. And if the lordosis is out of vicinity time and again or for extended periods or each, decrease once more issues generally take location.

ANATOMY

To recognize why lower returned issues may additionally arise from lack of the lordosis, permit's speedy have a have a have a look at human anatomy.

The human backbone is view from the aspect (Fig.2.2).

The backbone or "spine" (Fig. 2.2) is made from vertebrae. Each vertebra seems simply like a spool of thread (Fig. 2.Three). It is round and has a hole this is going from top to bottom.

There are thirty-three vertebrae: seven in the neck (the cervical vertebrae), twelve inside the pinnacle yet again (the thoracic vertebrae), 5 within the the lower returned (the lumbar vertebrae), 5 fused inside the sacrum (the sacral vertebrae), and 4 rudimentary vertebrae fused inside the coccyx (thecoccygeal vertebrae; the ones are the lowest part of the backbone and are the vestige of a tail). With the vertebrae lined up one atop the alternative, the holes shape the spinal canal (Fig. 2.4). Through this canal runs the package deal of nerves that extends from the head to the pelvis, the spinal wire.

Figure 2.Three: The vertebrae are similar to a stack of cotton spools.

Figure (2.Four) A vertebra

Figure 2.Five: Two vertebrae

Between each pair of vertebrae are two tiny apertures via which the left and proper spinal nerves break out the spinal canal (Fig. 2.Five). Among exclusive topics, those nerves supply electricity to the muscle tissue and provide to revel in to the pores and pores and skin. It is through the spinal nerves that you may manual movement and experience temperature, stress, and pain. These feelings aren't in fact common components of life; further they offer a natural alarm system: they assist you to recognise that a physiological shape goes to preserve a few damage or has already been injured. In the decrease phase of the backbone, components of the left and proper spinal nerves be part of to deliver the left and proper sciatic nerves, which service the legs. When those nerves are overwhelmed or infected, they will produce discomfort in the leg. The pain frequently is going beneath the knee. Pain going from the decrease all over again to under the the knee is called sciatica. Between the spool-like vertebrae are precise systems, referred to as discs, made from cartilage, a dense connective tissue capable of withstanding full-size strain.

In the human body, there are 3 forms of cartilage: hyaline cartilage, elastic cartilage, and fibrocartilage.

The type gift in the spine is fibrocartilage. Intervertebral discs are specific cartilage systems some of the vertebrae. Just as the vertebrae are similar to spools, the discs are similar to rubber washers, round, and shaped of a bendy substance; no longer like many washers, but, they do now not have a hollow inside the center.

The semifluid center of the disc is called the nucleus pulposus, "nucleus" for brief. Surrounding the nucleus is a cartilage ring, termed the annulus or annular ligament.

The discs are the surprise absorbers of the spine. They are bendy sufficient that they may alter their form, allowing one vertebra to slide on some other and allowing movement of the lower lower again as an entire.

The vertebrae and discs of the lower all over again compose the lumbar spine and are associated thru using severa joints. Each joint is held together thru easy tissues that surround it. These tissues are bolstered through ligaments, hard bands of fibrous connective tissue.

The ligaments that enhance the tablet that surrounds a spinal joint are like man wires that manual an outside television antenna through pulling on it and attaching it to the roof.

The spinal ligaments offer a lift to the the joint and restriction its mobility to precise hints. Then there are the muscle tissues, which lay over one or extra joints of the decrease again. The muscle tissue acquire upward to the trunk and downward to the pelvis. At each end, each muscle develops a tendon, which links the muscle to one or more bones. When a muscle contracts, it creates movement in one or more joints.

Back Pain Exercise:

Knee-to-chest stretch:

Do you want to prevent again ache? Try those physical games to stretch and red meat up your again and supporting muscular tissues. Repeat each exercising a few times, then growth the repetitions due to the fact the exercising receives lots much less complex.

Lie to your over again collectively collectively together with your knees bent and your toes flat on the ground (A). Using both palms, deliver up one leg and push it on your chest (B). Tighten your abdominals and push your backbone to the ground. Hold for 5 seconds. Return to the start feature and repeat with the opposing leg (C). Return to the start characteristic and then repeat with each legs on the identical time (D). Repeat every stretch 2 to a few times ideally as quickly as in the morning and once at night time.

Lower over again rotational stretch:

Lie to your back together together with your knees bent and your toes flat on the floor (A). Keeping your shoulders firmly on the floor, roll your bent knees to as a minimum one component (B). Hold for five to 10 seconds. Return to the start function (C). Repeat at the opportunity facet (D). Repeat each stretch 2 to a few times. Preferably once in the morning and once at night time.

Lower lower again flexibility exercising:

Lie to your all over again together together with your knees bent and your toes flat on the ground (A). Tighten your stomach muscle tissue so your belly pulls a long way from your waistband (B). Hold for 5 seconds and then loosen up. Flatten your again, pulling your belly button in the route of the ground (C). Hold for 5 seconds and then loosen up. Repeat. Start with 5 repetitions every day and regularly paintings as a great deal as 30.

Bridge workout:

Lie to your once more at the side of your knees bent and your ft flat at the ground (A). Keeping your shoulders and head relaxed at the floor, tighten your stomach and gluteal muscle groups. Then growth your hips to make a straight line from your knees on your shoulders (B). Try to maintain the posture prolonged enough to complete 3 deep breaths. Return to the begin location and repeat. Start with 5 repetitions every day and frequently paintings as plenty as 30.

Cat stretch

Position your self on your arms and knees (A). Slowly arch your decrease once more, as if you're pulling your belly up towards the ceiling (B). Then slowly permit your once more and stomach sag closer to the ground (C). Return to the start characteristic (A). Repeat 3 to 5 times two times a day.

Seated decrease decrease returned rotational stretch:

Sit on an armless chair or a stool. Cross your proper leg over your left leg. Bracing your left elbow in the direction of the out of doors of your proper knee, twist and stretch to the issue (A). Hold for 10 seconds. Repeat on the possibility side (B). Repeat this stretch 3 to 5 instances on each aspect two times a day.

Shoulder blade squeeze:

Sit on an armless chair or a stool (A). While preserving real posture, pull your shoulder blades collectively (B). Hold for 5 seconds and then lighten up. Repeat three to 5 instances times an afternoon.

COMMON BACK REMEDIES AND SOLUTIONS:

MEDICINES AND DRUGS

As noted earlier on this book, most of the commonplace again pains we revel in are mechanical in basis and therefore are affected simplest with the aid of the usage of the ones drugs and medicines that may relieve ache. There aren't any drugs or drugs able to put off the motives of our not unusual backaches and pains. Therefore, remedy need to be taken great whilst your pains are immoderate or while you need to discover alleviation. Certain medicinal capsules, together with aspirin and special nonsteroidal anti-inflammatory tablets (NSAIDs), are the most beneficial for alleviating acute all over again pain and characteristic fewer aspect effects than a few commonly prescribed medications. Both were advocated via the U.S. Government's Agency for Health Care Policy and Research (now the Agency for Healthcare Research and Quality).

BED REST

When your decrease once more ache is so severe that bed rest is vital, you want to limit this time of rest, if in any respect possible, to two or three days. A have a study completed within the United States established that sufferers who rested in bed for 2 days recovered in addition to folks who stayed in mattress for seven days. But patients who continued to walk and exercising were capable of pass again to paintings in advance than folks that slept for each or seven days.

ACUPUNCTURE

Acupuncture can relieve ache and, even as all else has failed, is properly sincerely truely really worth a attempt.

You need to be conscious, but, that as with taking medicinal tablets, acupuncture can offer you with remedy, but it can't correct the underlying mechanical trouble.

BACK PAIN IN THE COMMUNITY

Lower back pain is huge finally of the arena, each in Western and Eastern cultures. In Western international locations, wherein more statistics are available, approximately 80 percentage of people will at the least one time of their lives go through a again ache episode so severe as to require bed relaxation. Many topics may be completed to beautify this case. You as an character need to complain each time you find beside the factor seating in public offices or houses or public transit automobiles. If your vehicle's seats are inadequate, you have to bitch on your car provider; higher however, look for every other automobile or do not forget having your automobile retrofitted with higher seats.

I turned into approximately to put in writing, "When choosing residing room fixtures" but an American friend of mine has suggested me that inside the United States a "living room" is generally a bar or a ladies's restroom. So I will rephrase. I suggest to comment on furniture used for fun at home. So I will say that once choosing living room furnishings (which almost commonly appears designed to reason or perpetuate again issues), you have to persist until you find chairs which is probably properly designed. When you're in a furnishings shop and find out seating this is poorly designed, you ought to inform the manager that this is the case.

If you complain to a automobile dealer or a furnishings keep supervisor, nothing will alternate right away. But enough court cases can result in reform. Few airlines offer seating that thoroughly lets in the lower all over again. This has excessive results for some individuals who need to fly prolonged distances and for lots hours. Office employees need to call for seating that offers excellent enough lumbar manual. There are many sophisticated-looking and high-priced place of business and secretarial chairs in the marketplace that provide no lumbar help by any way.

On the opportunity hand, chairs that provide suitable beneficial aid can frequently be placed at slight fees. Although bad seating layout is a prime element contributing to the Although terrible seating layout is a first-rate element contributing to the improvement of lower once more pain, any other, more crucial element is becoming an increasing number of evident. Where as quickly as our faculty bodily training instructors were worried with poor posture in our children and corrected it when they noticed it, they now appear more interested by producing the exceptional soccer group, the very superb-scoring basketball player, and the quickest sprinter. Physical education teachers in all regions of the globe now not appear to offer our children with the records this is so vital if they're to take care of their bodily necessities over a whole life within the international.

Spinal ache of postural foundation might not emerge if this essential statistics have been given to human beings at an early age.

Ask any twelve-yr-vintage teen whether he or she has been taught at university a way to stand properly or a way to take a seat successfully. Chances are that the kid will permit you to recognise that she or he has in no way been shown both of these vital postures. Similarly, probabilities are slim that the child has been informed about the harmful outcomes which could upward thrust up if posture is overlooked. If the ones topics are of trouble to you, you would likely with courtesy request that your university management or P.E. Teachers make postural physical education a subject. In addition, you could advise that directors have a examine college furnishings for its effects on posture.

Good postural behavior must be instilled at an early age.

These are sports that you as a concerned individual may moreover do to help result in a number of the changes that need to arise if society is to have interaction rationally with the big hassle of once more ache. In the us by myself, this trouble expenses $50 to $70 billion a three hundred and sixty five days in everything from scientific charges to days misplaced from artwork.

Chapter 5: Rebuilding Hip Pain

The hip joint can hold repetitive motion and a significant diploma of damage and tear and tear and tear. This ball-and-socket joint the body's largest fits collectively in a manner that allows for easy movement.

Whenever you make use of the hip (as an example, via going for a run), a cushion of cartilage aids reduces friction due to the fact the hip bone rotates in its socket. Despite its staying power, the hip joint is not unbreakable. With age and utilization, the cartilage may furthermore put on out or get injured. Muscles and tendons of the hip ought to probable grow to be overworked. Bones inside the hip could likely shatter following a fall or amazing twist of destiny. Any of those problems may additionally cause hip pain. If your hips are hurting, proper here is an define of what may be inflicting your ache and the manner to acquire hip ache remedy.

Causes of Hip Pain

These are a number of the situations that usually purpose hip pain:

1. Arthritis.

Osteoarthritis and rheumatoid arthritis are the numerous most not unusual motives of hip discomfort, in particular in older individuals. Arthritis results in irritation of the hip joint and the destruction of the cartilage that cushions your hip bones. The ache finally grows worse. People with arthritis additionally revel in stiffness and feature a confined variety of motion inside the hip. Learn extra about hip osteoarthritis.

2. Hip fractures.

With growing vintage, the bones can also end up vulnerable. Weakened bones are more at risk of shatter in the path of a fall. Learn more about hip fracture signs and symptoms and signs and symptoms.

3. Bursitis.

Bursae are sacs of fluids positioned amongst tissues such as bone, muscle agencies, and tendons. They reduce the friction from those tissues rubbing collectively. When bursae develop infected, they'll purpose discomfort. Inflammation of the bursae is mainly associated with repeated actions that overwork or get worse the hip joint. Learn extra about bursitis of the hip.

four. Tendinitis.

Tendons are the thick bands of tissue that bind bones to muscle groups. Tendinitis is infection or irritation of the tendons. It's frequently attributable to repeated strain from usage. Learn extra approximately tendinitis signs and symptoms and signs.

five. Muscle or tendon strain.

Repeated sports activities sports may additionally additionally impose tension on the muscle businesses, tendons, and ligaments that useful resource the hips. When they come to be infected thanks to misuse, they may motive discomfort and hinder the hip from going for walks nicely. Learn approximately the incredible stretches for stiff hip muscle corporations.

6. Hip labral tear.

This is a tear inside the ring of cartilage (referred to as the labrum) that follows the outer rim of the socket of your hip joint. Along with cushioning your hip joint, your labrum abilities like a rubber seal or gasket to assist preserve the ball on the top of your thighbone firmly inner your hip socket. Athletes and all of us who executes repeated twisting motions are at elevated hazard of having this condition. Learn greater approximately hip labral tears.

7. Cancers.

Tumors that growth within the bone or that unfold to the bone may additionally additionally furthermore reason ache inside the hips, further to in different bones of the frame. Learn greater approximately bone tumors. Avascular necrosis (from time to time termed osteonecrosis). This hassle arises at the same time as the blood supply to the hip bone decreases and the bone tissue dies. Although it can have an effect on other bones, avascular necrosis most normally develops in the hip. It can be because of a hip fracture or dislocation, or thru the lengthy-time period use of excessive-dose steroids (together with prednisone), amongst specific motives.

Symptoms of Hip Pain

Depending on the situation this is causing your hip pain, you may experience pain in your:

Thigh

Inside of the hip joint

Groin

Outside of the hip joint

Buttocks

Sometimes ache from excellent components of the body, which incorporates the once more or groin (from a hernia), can also radiate to the hip. You need to find that your ache grows worse with workout, specifically if it's because of arthritis. Along with the ache, you could have a limited type of motion. Some humans acquire a limp from extended hip ache.

Hip Pain Relief

If your hip pain is because of a muscle or tendon strain, osteoarthritis, or tendinitis, you could typically ease it with an over-the-counter pain medicinal drug which incorporates acetaminophen or a nonsteroidal anti inflammatory drug which consist of ibuprofen or naproxen. Rheumatoid arthritis treatment alternatives moreover embody prescription anti-inflammatory capsules consisting of corticosteroids, ailment-improving anti-rheumatic capsules (DMARDs) like methotrexate and sulfasalazine, and biologics, which target the immune tool.

Another way to relieve hip ache is thru preserving ice to the location for about 15 minutes some instances an afternoon. Try to relaxation the affected joint as an entire lot as possible till you experience higher. You also can moreover attempt heating the vicinity. A warm temperature bath or bathe can help prepared your muscle for stretching sports activities that might lessen pain. If you have were given have been given arthritis, exercise the hip joint with low-effect sporting events, stretching, and resistance education can reduce pain and beautify joint mobility. For example, swimming is a great non-impact workout for arthritis. Physical remedy also can assist increase your range of motion.

When osteoarthritis will become so immoderate that the ache is excessive or the hip joint becomes deformed, a complete hip substitute (arthroplasty) may be a interest. People who fracture their hip every now and then need surgical operation to repair the fracture or replace the hip. Call your healthcare issuer in case your ache doesn't depart, or in case you phrase swelling, redness, or warm temperature throughout the joint. Also, call when you have hip ache at night time or while you are resting.

Get medical help proper away if:

The hip pain came on .

A fall or one of a kind damage precipitated the hip pain.

Your joint seems deformed or are bleeding.

You heard a popping noise in the joint even as you injured it.

The ache is intense.

You can't located any weight for your hip.

You can not flow your leg or hip.

Exercises and stretches for hip ache:

There are many feasible reasons of hip pain, beginning from muscle lines and injuries to arthritis and inflammatory problems. However, gently workout the hips can frequently assist relieve pain and repair mobility. In this positioned up, we speak 8 sports sports which can help beautify the hips, decorate joint mobility, and reduce hip discomfort.

Considerations earlier than beginning

Flexibility and energy sports activities sports are important to alleviating hip pain. Although those exercising workouts may bring about quick pain, they want to now not purpose or worsen the ache. If an interest motives pain, forestall performing it or try continuing at a slower or softer speed. Individuals who've presently passed through a hip replacement should go to a scientific medical doctor or bodily therapist earlier than challenge any of the sports sports beneath.

Exercises 1–four

The first four sports activities stretch the muscle organizations throughout the hip joint, that may help reduce stiffness and beautify joint mobility. A person should perform the ones bodily video video games at times even as they are feeling the least amount of pain and stiffness. A nicely time to do them is after a heat bathe or bathtub even as the muscle organizations are maximum snug. Begin with one or physical video games a day, three instances each week. If this appears snug, bear in mind finishing numerous sporting activities as quickly as a day.

Exercises five–8

The purpose of these workout exercises is to reinforce the hip muscle tissue to higher help the hip joint, which may additionally assist reduce pain. Resistance schooling is a form of exercising for boosting muscular electricity. In resistance schooling, a person makes use of both slight weights or body mass to deliver resistance for their muscle agencies to art work towards. People who've hip pain or soreness for added than an hour after those sporting activities must lower the significant variety of repetitions effectively.

1. Knee increase.

To execute knee lifts:

Lie on the another time, stretching each legs flat down the ground.

Keeping the left leg at once, pull the proper knee up within the direction of the chest.

Place each fingers on top of the knee to gently deliver it in toward the chest.

Hold the stretch for 10 seconds.

Let go of the knee and little by little drop the leg decrease decrease returned in the route of the floor.

Repeat this exercising five–10 instances on each knee.

2. External hip rotation.

To accomplish external hip rotations:

Sit on the floor with every legs out in the front.

Bend the legs at the knees and squeeze the soles of the feet together.

Place a hand on top of each knee and lightly push them every down inside the route of the ground. Apply stress to the knees until there may be a stretch, however do not push them in addition than is snug.

Hold the stretch for 10 seconds and then lighten up.

Repeat the stretch five–10 instances.

3. Double hip rotation.

To execute double hip rotations:

Lie down at the yet again. Then, bend the knees and pull them inside the course of the body till the feet are flat on the floor.

Gently twist the knees to the left, reducing them within the route of the floor. Rotate the head to stand the right at the same time as preserving the shoulders in opposition to the floor.

Hold this posture for 20–30 seconds.

Slowly go back each the pinnacle and knees to the beginning feature.

Repeat at the opportunity aspect.

4. Hip and lower again stretch.

To execute hip and decrease yet again stretches:

Lying flat on the decrease back, bend the knees and pull them within the course of the frame till the toes are level at the floor.

Using the arms, draw each knees in toward the chest.

Breathe deeply, pulling the knees closer to the shoulders with each exhalation.

Go as some distance as is snug, then maintain the area for 20–30 seconds. Breathe usually.

5. Hip flexion.

To carry out hip flexions:

Stand upright.

Extend one arm out to the factor and hold on to a sturdy floor, collectively with a wall, table, or chair, for assist.

Slowly increase the proper knee to the quantity of the hip or as a protracted way as is snug on the equal time as maintaining the left leg proper away.

Only keep this role for a 2d in advance than placing the left foot once more at the ground.

Repeat with the left knee.

Do five–10 repetitions of this exercise.

6. Hip extension.

To carry out hip extensions:

Stand erect with the legs without delay and the feet shoulder-width aside.

Extend each palms out inside the the front and hold on to a chair, desk, or wall for help.

Keeping the right leg immediately, improve the left leg backward with out bending the knee.

Lift the leg as a long manner as viable without growing pain, then clench the buttock strongly and preserve the posture for 5 seconds.

Repeat this stretch 5–10 times on every leg. To increase the resistance, try attaching small weights to the legs.

7. Hip abduction.

To carry out hip abduction sporting activities:

Stand upright.

Extend the left arm out to the issue and maintain without delay to three issue strong, which includes a chair, desk, or wall.

Starting with the ft collectively, carry the right leg out to the right component. Keep the left leg instantly and avoid rotating the hips.

Hold the location for five seconds after which slowly skip once more the leg to the start position.

Do this exercise 5–10 instances on one leg, then repeat it on the opportunity thing.

eight. Heal to buttocks exercising

To execute heel-to-buttock bodily sports:

Stand erect with the legs right away and the ft shoulder-width aside. For guide, keep directly to a chair, desk, or wall.

Bending the left knee, supply the heel up closer to the left buttock with the pinnacle of the foot handling the ground. Be sure to preserve the right leg instantly and align the knees.

Slowly decrease the leg and pass again to the beginning characteristic.

Repeat the workout on the opportunity side.

Aim to do 5–10 repetitions on each leg.

Chapter 6: Healing Knee And Ankle Problem

Have you latterly suffered from an ankle or knee sprain? One day you're lively and capable to stroll/run successfully and the following, you're having terrible soreness originating from your knee or ankle. After a entire examination, you are recognized with an ankle or knee sprain. The venture now could be, how do you get better?

WHAT IS A SPRAIN?

Every joint within the body incorporates bands of tissue that maintain the joint together. These bands are known as ligaments. When the ligaments flip outdoor of their conventional form of motion, inflicting them to overstretch or rupture, the disorder has termed a sprain. In ankles, the ligaments at the outside of the joint are the maximum susceptible to harm. In the knees, any of the ligaments might be torn for the cause that knee rotates in numerous outstanding pointers.

Causes of Knee and Ankle Pain:

There are severa motives for ache within the knee, foot, and ankle. Some of the motives are:

Sprains

Injuries or fracture

Overuse of the muscle tissues

Dislocations

Arthritis, gout, bursitis, tendonitis, or precise comparable conditions

Infection

Weight benefit

Nerve damage

Tumors

THE THREE PHASES OF RECOVERY

Every ankle sprain or knee sprain has 3 tiers of restoration. While restoration takes amongst weeks and months, there may be no secret recipe for making the approach waft faster. However, continuously working thru those stages allows the joint to heal correctly and lowers the possibility of re-injuring the joint.

PHASE 1: RICE.

The initial phase of joint rehabilitation can be summarized with the acronym RICE - Rest, Ice, Compression, Elevation. This segment would probable growth from some days, as a brilliant deal as each week to allow the ankle or knee an possibility to start recuperation.

Rest your knee or ankle with the useful resource of keeping off strolling or strolling on it, using crutches if required.

Ice the knee or ankle for 20 minutes at a time to hold infection at a minimum. However, you need to by no means examine ice without delay at the pores and pores and skin. Instead, wrap an ice percent in a moderate towel or pillowcase to keep away from frostbite.

Compression can be finished via using a brace or wrap at the damage. Not only does compression offer aid to a weaker joint, but it decreases edema as properly.

Elevating the knee or ankle above the waist or the coronary coronary heart furthermore lowers edema inside the joint. Prop it up on cushions, the arm of the sofa, or any strong, mild floor.

PHASE 2: INCREASE FLEXIBILITY & RANGE OF MOTION.

Once the swelling has started out out to lessen, you are equipped to undertake the subsequent section of recuperation - enhancing flexibility and range of motion in the joint. At this point, enlisting the assist of a bodily therapist can assist restore power and balance in your knee or ankle at the same time as reducing the threat of re-injuring it inside the method. A bodily therapist may additionally moreover do move friction rubdown that assures the ligaments will no longer inappropriately maintain to the bone.

PT at this level moreover includes severa palms-on remedies that maintain to decrease edema and control pain with out the want for heavy dosages of ache capsules.

PHASE 3: RESTORE STRENGTH & BALANCE.

Once the joint has all started out out to heal, a physical therapist can then prescribe strengthening bodily activities as a way to assist restore your form of motion, energy, stability, and proprioception (the ability to enjoy wherein the joint is in area). Many humans expect that after they're now not in pain, they will pass lower again to regular sports activities sports. In fact, physical remedy is the handiest way a person can achieve an entire healing from a knee or ankle sprain. A cautiously constructed, supervised exercising software program application not handiest permits to reinforce the ligaments maintaining the joint collectively, however it moreover strengthens the muscle companies all through the joint, stopping destiny accidents. When carried out efficaciously, with bodily remedy, getting higher from a knee or ankle sprain can go away you as actual as new in a few short weeks. Always searching for recommendation from your bodily therapist or physician earlier than starting sports activities activities you're unsure of doing.

Chapter 7: How To Be Relief From Shoulder Pain

Shoulder soreness is any pain in or across the shoulder joint.

Considerations:

The shoulder is the maximum movable joint within the human frame. A set of 4 muscle tissues and related tendons, termed the rotator cuff, offer the shoulder a brilliant type of movement. Swelling, damage, or bone adjustments surrounding the rotator cuff may moreover reason shoulder pain. You may moreover revel in discomfort at the same time as raising the arm over your head or transferring it forward or within the decrease again of your lower back.

Causes

The most not unusual purpose of shoulder pain arises while rotator cuff tendons get trapped underneath the bony place of the shoulder. The tendons become indignant or injured. This state of affairs is called rotator cuff tendinitis or bursitis.

Shoulder ache can also be because of:

Arthritis in the shoulder joint.

Bone spurs within the shoulder region.

Bursitis is inflammation of a fluid-stuffed sac (bursa) that typically protects the joint and enables it skip without problems.

Broken shoulder bone.

Dislocation of the shoulder.

Shoulder separation.

Frozen shoulder, which takes vicinity at the equal time as the muscle tissues, tendons, and ligaments in the shoulder turn out to be inflexible, making movement tough and ugly Overuse or harm of neighboring tendons, which includes the bicep muscle corporations of the palms.

Nerve harm that results in atypical shoulder motion.

Tears of the rotator cuff tendons.

Poor shoulder posture and mechanics.

Shoulder joint dislocation.

This animation indicates dislocation of the shoulder joint.

Sometimes, shoulder pain can be connected to a situation in some other a part of the body, which incorporates the neck or lungs. This is referred to as referred pain. There is commonly pain at relaxation and no worsening of ache even as shifting the shoulder.

Home Care

Here are a few hints for helping shoulder pain get better:

Put ice on the shoulder region for 15 minutes, then leave it off for 15 minutes. Do this 3 to four instances a day for 2 to 3 days. Wrap the ice in material. Do now not located ice straight away at the pores and pores and skin due to the fact this will result in frostbite.

Rest your shoulder for the subsequent few days.

Slowly flow lower back to your everyday sports activities activities. A bodily therapist will permit you to do that successfully.

Taking ibuprofen or acetaminophen (at the side of Tylenol) may additionally additionally help decrease irritation and discomfort.

Rotator cuff problems can be addressed at domestic as well:

If you have got have been given skilled shoulder problem previously, make use of ice and ibuprofen after exercising.

Learn bodily video games to stretch and provide a boost for your rotator cuff tendons and shoulder muscle tissues. A medical health practitioner or bodily therapist may additionally prescribe such physical games.

If you are becoming better from tendinitis, hold to adopt variety-of-motion sporting occasions to prevent a frozen shoulder.

Practice proper posture to preserve your shoulder muscle tissues and tendons in their appropriate locations.

When to Contact a Medical Professional

Sudden left shoulder pain can once in a while be a sign of a coronary heart attack. Call 911 or your neighborhood emergency big variety when you have sudden stress or crushing ache for your shoulder, specifically if the pain runs from your chest to the left jaw, arm, or neck, or takes vicinity with shortness of breath, dizziness, or sweating. Go to the hospital emergency room when you have truly had a excessive damage and your shoulder can be very painful, swollen, bruised, or bleeding.

Call your fitness care company when you have:

Shoulder ache with a fever, swelling, or redness.

Problems moving the shoulder.

Pain for greater than 2 to 4 weeks, even after home remedy.

Swelling of the shoulder.

.Red or blue shade of the pores and pores and skin of the shoulder region

Chapter 8: Osteoporosis Defined

Osteoporosis is a disease that occurs because of lessening bone density. This lessening happens slowly and progressively for years without any signs or symptoms. That is why osteoporosis often said as a silent disease. The symptoms will show up when the disease becomes worse, such as bone fracture, hunch back, losing body height, and back pain. About 80 % of osteoporosis patients are women. It has a correlation with the fact that women are having menopause that cause them losing estrogen, a hormone with a function to save calcium to the bone. But men can also suffer from osteoporosis. One of five men above 50 year-old suffers from this disease.

Causes and Risk Factors of Osteoporosis

What is the actual cause of osteoporosis?

Some factors play role in causing this disease. Here are they:

1.   Postmenopausal   osteoporosis.   This happens because of decrease of estrogen, the main gonad hormone in a woman which has a function to store calcium to the bone.

2. Senile osteoporosis, possibly because of lack of calcium intake during life. It has a correlation with age and imbalance of bone destruction and formation.

3. Secondary osteoporosis, caused by other medical condition or by drug induced. Osteoporosis may be caused by chronic kidney disease, hiperparathyroidism, long use of corticosteroids, barbiturates, etc. Alcohol abuse and smoking may worsen osteoporosis.

4. Juvenile idiopathic osteoporosis, a kind of osteoporosis with unknown cause. It attacks children and teenager with normal hormone level and function, normal vitamin and no exact cause of bone fragility.

These are the risk factors:

1. Woman. It has a correlation with the decrease of estrogen (start from age 35) and menopause.

2. Age. The older you are, the bigger the chance of having osteoporosis.

3. Race. The white and the Asian have the highest risk. It is commonly because of the low consumption of calcium of

Asian women. African and Hispanic have lower risks.

4. Family history of osteoporosis.

If one of your relatives has an osteoporosis you have to be careful. Osteoporosis attacks people with specific bone character, such as same bone structure in a family.

5. Bad lifestyle, includes:

Excessive consumption of red meat and soft drinks. Both of them contain phosphor that may stimulate the secretion of parathyroid hormone which causes release of calcium from bone to blood.

Caffeine and alcohol. They may cause bone fragile and damaged. Urine of one consuming caffeine or alcohol contains more calcium that comes from bone destruction. Besides, caffeine and alcohol is toxic which inhibit formation of bone mass.

Lazy doing sport. One who is lazy to move or to do sport will cause inhibition of osteoblastic process. Movements and sports are good stimulation to bone formation. Lazy to move will also decrease bone density.

Smoking. Nicotine can stimulate bone resorption. It also decreases estrogen level and activity.

Low blood calcium level. It will cause the body to secrete hormones that cause the blood takes calcium from other parts of the body including the bones.

6. Drug consumption. Corticosteroids used by asthma and allergic patients may inhibit bone formation. Heparin and anti-seizure drugs

may do the same. Consult to your doctor before using this kind of drug.

7. Thin and tiny. This body posture tends to make body lighter. Bones are diligent to form cells if they are pressed by heavy bodyweight. So, thin and tiny people have the higher risk to suffer from osteoporosis.

Diagnosing Osteoporosis

If someone, for example a 70 year-old lady has shown a symptom of osteoporosis such as bone fracture, the diagnosis of osteoporosis will be confirmed based on the signs and symptoms she has been experienced. The physician will also ask whether she has the risk factors of osteoporosis.

Then he/she will do some physical examination and an x-ray examination. Other examinations may be needed to know another possibility of the fracture.

The Osteoporosis Therapy

Therapy and medication of osteoporosis has a goal to increase bone density, to lessen extra-fracture, and to control the pain. To determine the best therapy includes multidisciplinary aspects. A

team from surgery department, internal department, obstetric and gynecology department will be involved. A clinical nutritionist should also be consulted.

The therapy will be given appropriate with the patient's need. If there is a bone fracture the doctor will examine whether it needs a surgical treatment or a splinting. After that, the patient should take physiotherapy to rehabilitate the bone ability.

The pharmacological treatment will be needed to prevent another fracture. This can be given to the patient who has not experienced fracture but has osteoporosis, for example from a screening. Here are the drugs:

1. Biphosphonate.

This drug is useful to prevent bone damage, to restore bone mass, and to increase bone density especially of the back and the hip. Drugs include in this group are risendronate, alendronate, pamidronate, chlodronate, zoledronate (zoledronic acid), and ibandronic acid.

2. Selective estrogen receptor modulator (SERM).

It is a kind of hormone replacement therapy for a postmenopausal woman. It is effective to decrease bone turnover and to slow the resorption of bone mass. An example of SERM is raloxifene.

3. Vitamin D metabolites that is calcitriol and alpha calcidol.

They have ability to help body absorbing calcium.

4. Calcitonin.

This drug is suggested to someone who had spine fracture with pain. This drug can be injected or can be given by nasal spray.

5. Strontium Ranelate.

This drug improves bone formation by activating osteoblast and by forming collagen and also decrease bone resoprtion by lowering osteoclast activity.

Osteoporosis Prevention

Osteoporosis is a disease wherein bones become fragile or porous and thus brittle, leading to easy fractures. A bone mineral density test (BMD) is the only way one can diagnose osteoporosis and thus determine any risks for future fracture. The main reason BMD has to be done is because osteoporosis can go It is through this that one determines if treatment is needed to maintain bone mass and prevents further bone loss.

The best defense against osteoporosis is building strong bones, especially before the age of thirty, and maintaining a healthy lifestyle. However, although there are treatments for osteoporosis, there is no actual cure for it. There are

five steps for preventing osteoporosis, which have to be adapted jointly to help prevent osteoporosis. First of all, the daily recommended amounts of calcium and vitamin D must be consumed for the heart, muscles and nerves to function properly, and for blood to clot.

Inadequate calcium highly contributes to the development of osteoporosis. So 1,000 and 1,300 mg of calcium has to be consumed daily, from the foods you eat or through calcium supplements.

Vitamin D is needed for the body to absorb calcium and is available through the skin from direct exposure to sunlight and from foods like liver and egg yolks.

Maintain a regular weight-bearing exercise routine, like walking, dancing, jogging and racquet sports, to get good bone health. You are more likely to reach your peak bone density if you exercise regularly in childhood and adolescence. It is also better to avoid smoking and consumption of excessive alcohol to prevent osteoporosis. Although there is no actual cure for osteoporosis, bisphosphonates, calcitonin, parathyroid hormone, estrogens and raloxifene are approved for the prevention of osteoporosis. Of course, the best thing to do to prevent the onset of osteoporosis is to have a bone density test and to take appropriate medication.

How to Prevent and Treat Osteoporosis

Osteoporosis is a common health hazard especially for women over 50 even though men run a moderately strong risk of developing the disease as well. There is a plethora of information available today that can cause confusion as to how to prevent or limit the progression of the disease before it causes serious damage to bones. While there are many things that you can do to help prevent osteoporosis, the short answer is that the disease can be prevented by building stronger bones before the age of 30. This is the best prevention against the disease in later life. Although, there are several things you can do later on that will also help resist the onset of the disease or the progression of it if you have already been diagnosed. Since osteoporosis is an often complicated disease, it requires not just one preventive health protocol, but rather several.

#1 - You must ingest the recommended amount of vitamin D and calcium.

Vitamin D is critical for the proper absorption of calcium in the body to take place. If your body does not have enough vitamin D to process calcium in your body, then your body will slowly remove the necessary vitamin D from your bones in order to synthesize the calcium. Vitamin D is absorbed into the body through two methods: through the sun and through the diet. If you're under 50, you need a daily dosage of 400-800 IU's and if you're over 50, you need to take at least between 800-1,000 IU's daily for proper calcium absorption.

The D vitamin is also found in foods such as egg yolks, liver, and saltwater dish.

#2 - In order to create the proper body balance for fighting osteoporosis, you should abstain from smoking altogether as well as indulging in excessive alcohol. As in many other health issues, osteoporosis is only exacerbated by these negative health activities and puts users at a higher risk for the disease later in life.

#3 - Add a fitness regimen that includes weight bearing exercises at least 3 or 4 days a week for best results.

Exercises such as jogging, walking, climbing stairs, and hiking are good, basic activities.

Sports such as tennis and racuetball are also good fitness activities. If you are training at a gym, the addition of lighter weight lifting exercises are very helpful for strengthening the hip joints and spine. If you have never included weight lifting in your fitness workout, you may benefit from the expertise of a trainer for a while as you learn the basic uses of weight equipment and how to exercise the correct body areas. A balanced approach to fitness is always best by mixing up both cardio and weight bearing exercises.

#4 - Be sure to talk to your healthcare professional about your bone health as well as undergo bone density testing whenever your healthcare provider suggests it. Usually those over 50 should begin to watch for any bone thinning and deterioration. Your doctor can prescribe various types of medication that can also help prevent bone loss if you are at risk.

Be sure to actively combat your risk for osteoporosis not only after the age of 50 but well before, if possible. However, if you find that your are now at risk for developing the disease or are already showing signs of bone thinning, you can still follow these sensible

and practical   suggestions on combating or
slowing further development of osteoporosis.

Chapter 9: Exercise And Osteoporosis

The human body has 206 bones that are continually renewing themselves through a process known as remodeling. Bone cells called osteoclasts break existing bone down and remove it, while osteoblasts work in the other way and are responsible for depositing new bone. A persons maximum bone density will be achieved between the ages of 20 to 30. After this point osteoclast and osteoblast activity will remain in balance until around the age of 45 to 50, when osteoclast activity will become greater and the person will start to slowly lose bone mass.

People most at risk of Osteoporosis are:

Elderly - the older an individual, the greater the risk of osteoporosis, caused by the deteriorating effects after 45 to 50. Females - females are four times more likely than males to develop osteoporosis. This is due to the fact that they generally start with a lower peak bone mass than males, and will experience a sharp loss in bone mass following menopause.

Small Boned and Thin Women - due to a lack of bone bearing weight during their everyday lives. Lifestyle - smoking, drinking too much alcohol, drinking more than two cups of coffee per day, performing insufficient weight bearing exercise, and a diet lacking in calcium will all increase your chances of developing osteoporosis. To strengthen your bones you must directly target them in your workouts, making sure every part of your body is covered in your session. Exercises chosen should be weight bearing. Swimming and cycling are great for the cardiovascular system, but they place little stress on the bones. Walking and running are good aerobic activities to perform and of course weight training provides greatest benefits. Weight training should be performed at least twice a week to gain a benefit.

Training should be specific with each bone directly involved in the session. Working the leg muscles will not provide any benefit to the upper body.

For the bone to improve its density it must be stressed beyond its normal limits. If you are performing an exercise easily then the weight you are using is too light and must be increased. The bone will only adapt to the level that it is being worked at. Many females avoid heavy weights, fearful of putting on large amounts of muscle. This fear is misplaced however as females lack certain hormones that make it very hard for them to gain muscle mass. While it is important to build strong bones while we are young, it is never too late to start. No matter what age you are at, it is always possible to make an improvement. Weight training in the elderly will improve bone density, increase muscle mass and improve balance, reducing the risk of falling.

Weight training for elderly participants differs slightly, and should start slowly and gradually build up, always remaining in a relatively comfortable zone.

Weight training should be an integral part of every persons training regime, with a minimum of two sessions per week to gain the re?uired benefits.

Weight training is extremely important in combating the effects of osteoporosis, particularly for women and the elderly.

By completing regular resistance training sessions you will be laying a foundation for stronger, healthier bones and avoiding many of the potential dangers of old age.

Exercises for Healthy Bones

All forms of physical activity will help keep your bones strong and healthy and reduce the risk of falling. Check out the government's physical activity recommendations for:

children under 5 years

children and young people

adults

older adults

Physical activity is only 1 of the building blocks for strong, healthy bones – the others being eating food for healthy bones and avoiding certain risk factors for osteoporosis.

Children and Young People

Childhood, adolescence and early adulthood, when the skeleton is growing, are the time for building healthy bones. Children and young people should take part in moderate-to-vigorous intensity physical activity for an average of at least 60 minutes a day across the week.

Infants (less than 1 year)

Examples of muscle and bone- strengthening activities include:

tummy time

active play

crawling

Under 5s (walking)

Examples of muscle and bone- strengthening activities include:

climbing

walking

jumping

running

Children and Young People (up to 18 years old)

Examples of bone-strengthening activities include:

gymnastics

football

jumping

martial arts

Adults (over 19 years old)

Most muscle-strengthening or resistance exercise improves bone health. Do it at least 2 days a week.

Examples of activities for adults include:

circuit or resistance training

aerobics

ball games

tennis or racＺuet sports

running

dance

Older Adults

Examples of activities for active older adults include:

walking

lifting weights or using resistance bands

some impact activities like running, jumping or skipping

If you're not very active, these activities may help:

walking

stair climbing

strength exercises at home

To reduce the chance of falls, older adults are recommended to include activities that help with balance at least 2 days a week. For example:

tai chi

bowls

dance

Chapter 10: People With Osteoporosis

If you have osteoporosis or fragile bones, regular physical activity can help keep your bones healthy and reduce the risk of a fracture in the future. Depending on your risk of fracture, you may need to avoid some types of high- impact exercise. But if you're otherwise fit and healthy and already enjoy regular exercise, you should be able to continue.

Exercising And The Aging Process

Exercising becomes trickier as we age because, as our bodies change, the way they respond to different workouts changes as well. This difficulty is exacerbated by the need to work around different health conditions and chronic illnesses that plague us as we get older.

Below is a guide to exercising with health conditions that will allow you combat their negative effects on your health and maintain your exercise regimen in the face of disease.

1. Peripheral vascular disease (PVD)

It's important to exercise often with PVD to the point where exercising up to three times a day can be helpful. Avoid cold weather and cold water and slowly build your regimen up in intensity. Start out without using weights and instead perform exercises like swimming, rowing and cycling. Rest frequently and especially take care of your feet.

2. Lower back pain.

Many of us experience lower back pain when we age but it's possible to workout around this pain. Simply avoid hyperextension, non-supported supine flexion and the lifting of both legs in a supine or prone position. Do low-weight, high-rep exercises and make sure you stop if you feel pain.

3. Arthritis.

It's possible to cope with arthritis in the gym by performing longer warm-ups, exercising in a warm temperature and performing range of motion exercises every day. Also, practice isometric exercises and non-weight bearing exercises. Avoid cold temperatures.

4. Hypertension.

Exercising with hypertension is simple and it's just important to remember to breath properly during your exercises don't hold your breath - and avoid isometric exercises. Try to workout 4 times a week in 30 to 60 minute sessions.

5. Diabetes.

You might not think that diabetes has much impact on your workout but it's important to keep a few things in mind.

First, don't exercise when you blood sugar is too low (less than 100m/dl) or too high (greater than 300m/dl). Try to exercise within an hour of eating at roughly the same time every day. Also, try to workout 4 to 7 times a week in 40 to 60 minute sessions.

6. Osteoporosis.

It's possible to exercise around osteoporosis but it's important to avoid certain activity. Don't engage in any high impact aerobics, any sideways movements, movements that cross the midline of the body or spinal flexion.

Take part in resistance training and low impact aerobics such as walking or using an elliptical at least 4 times a week in 40 to 60 minute sessions.

The relationship between exercise and ageing isn't entirely about the interaction of health conditions and workouts but it is something important to keep in mind.

The above illnesses shouldn't keep you from working out and, as long as you follow these guidelines, you should be able to exercise without any issue.

When you have age-related health conditions, it's important to talk to an expert such as a personal trainer before working out. Such experts can instruct you in the proper techniques to use and can counsel you as to which exercises to avoid and which to engage in. Such experts are essential resources as we age and continue to exercise. Weight bearing exercise literally means the activity that puts your bones to bear your body weight. Although our bones always bear it the activity induces positive stress which helps the bone mineralisation and lowers bone loss. Weight Bearing Exercises for Osteoporosis prevention and cure:

Strength Training - If you have read this guide from the beginning you must have noticed my emphasis on strength training exercise. I am pro strength training not because it gives you a chiseled look but because metabolically you couldn't have asked for a better gift.

Strength training exercises that bear weight are low - medium intensity squats (with or without add on weights), same goes for lunges however please make sure you are accompanied by a trainer in order to correct your form during the exercise as squats and lunges if done in incorrect posture can do you harm than good. Leg extension and hamstring curl are another form of strength training exercise that allow weight bearing also good for building strength in the muscles around your knee and why is that so good for osteoporosis? Well matter of factly the knees bear the weight partially of the lower body next to the lower spine, so if your knees are strong they can afford to bear weight better. Hyper- extension of the back can also be good for the spinal bones strengthing the back muscles too, wrist flexion is also a good strength training exercise. The focus of these exercises I just mentioned is to firstly impact your hip, femur, tibia, wrist bones and spinal bones where osteoporosis is majorly seen. Strength training can also be done without any add on weights and that is what I personally practise too. You can do all the above exercises with the help of your own body weight with a little more intensity added to it. The use of terra bands, tubes, physio ball, water workouts for these exercises has turned out extremely beneficial.

Cardio Exercises - Walking is the best of all the options and it is absolutely possible wherever in the world you are with a good pair of shoes of course.

Walking puts adequate weight on the bones to impact on the reduction of bone loss. Similarly medium intensity elliptical trainer is also good as is climbing the stairwell to your apartment instead of the elevator. In fact climbing stairwell has proved to be a very good alternative in times when you cannot go out for a walk but need to continue exercising just keep your posture erect. Likewise swimming and water aerobics have benefits however these are more helpful during immediate rehabilitation after a fracture secondary to osteoporosis.

Yoga - The good old yoga proves to be a good weight bearing alternative but there are some asanas where you bend forward your turn your spine which would go against the idea of preventing osteoporosis, so don't attempt those positions.

Stretching - What you need to lower bone loss is have good weight impact on your spine and lower body bones with an erect posture. Joints where osteoporosis is fre?uent are hip, wrist, spine and if these are not flexible enough or let's just say are stiff your core muscles

(abdominal and lower back) will pull you forward giving a hunch back look and that's no good news for your spine bones which are already under stress of low bone mineral density and compression fractures. Stretching will free the joints and help attain a good posture and balance to the body keeping the add on stress on these bones at bay.

Great Reasons To Indulge In Lifelong Exercise

Many times you've read and heard the fact that exercising has a direct effect on your body and overall health. Here is a list of benefits gained by simply indulging in lifelong exercising.

Experience better sleep

If you didn't know, let me tell you that exercising helps you sleep well. People over the age of forty years often face problems with getting a good night sleep. Insomnia related issues can be solved with proper exercises.

Less tension and stress

With the hectic juggle of work and family, stress is an inevitable part of our lives. Doctors often recommend exercising as a cure to relieve stress. Your mind gets diverted from stressful matters and before you know it, the stress simply disappears.

Enjoy the fruits in the form of a healthy body

Exercising will help you maintain a healthy body weight. Obesity is a major concern in today's society, but if you exercise regularly, obesity will never be an issue.

Experience better performance and tolerance

Exercising has been proven to increase stamina and endurance. It also provides a better sense of well being which in turn increases tolerance towards things that would normally anger you.

Improves flexibility

Regular exercise loosens muscle and improves elasticity of the joints.

More Benefits

Exercising has some protective benefits as well. People who exercise daily face less number of strokes and heart attacks. Also, problems like hypertension, diabetes, obesity, depression and osteoporosis takes a back seat for those exercising on a regular basis. Taking part in aerobic exercise decreases blood pressure; strengthens the heart and improves blood flow.

Get Started!

Now that you are ready to get into the world of exercise and fitness, you need to decide on the best place to start your journey. Most people will locate a nearby workout facility, however there are many things you can do at home. Start with the basics such as sit-ups, pushups, jumping jacks and running in place. With exercising, you will also want to make some changes in your eating patterns so that you are able to maintain the body that exercising gifts you. If you are one that needs a push, look for a personal trainer, but choose a trainer who can help you decide what exercises are best for what you are trying to accomplish. In no time flat, you will notice a major difference in the way you look and feel. Good luck and have fun!

8 Core Benefits of Exercising

To keep active and healthy exercise is the best solution. Exercise is a solution to many problems and exercise helps to cure many diseases that may be more lethal if not taken care of. It helps the individuals to be active and more responsive though out the day.

Exercising daily makes you more fit and helps you avoid many diseases and illnesses. Here are some of the core befts of exercising:

1. It helps you to control your sugar level and hence avoid the chances of diabetes. It helps to promote healthy sugar level in your blood. It controls the sugar in your blood stream, which may not be possible otherwise. Controlling the sugar level by the means of daily exercise is much more effective than even using any medicine or even under any medical treatment. Controlling the sugar level with the help of exercise has no side effects.

2. It helps to strengthen your bones along with promoting the bone density. Bone density in turn helps to protect against the osteoporosis.

3. Exercising daily reduce the risk of many deadly diseases which principally include cancer. It helps to safeguard the individuals against many different cancers.

4. It helps the immune system of the individuals to be even stronger than before. It helps the individuals to protect against many minor diseases. If the immune system of a person is not very effective or strong he may

catch minor illnesses very quickly. So the exercise helps the individual to stay off those minor diseases.

5. It helps to increase the HDL level in the body and it helps to reduce the risk of heart attacks and many other heart related problems and complications.

6. It helps to lower the blood pressure which helps to reduce the risk factor that leads to heart attack.

7. It also helps to boost the self confidence of an individual, which helps him to avid depression and many else mental complications. It makes the individual to feel more confident and helps him to do the work that he may not be able to do in an ordinary condition.

8. Exercise when carried out with a good and balanced diet can help you gain weight and increase you muscle size for a better body shape and a healthier look. It helps you maintain a good body shape and helps you to

look more impressive. These were some of the core benefits of carrying out exercises at daily basis with regular workout and you can experience the difference with in no time. You just need to have a regular exercise routine and you can surely rock!

Chapter 11: Exercises For Osteoporosis

With age women suffer from osteoporosis, a condition where bones become weak due to calcium depletion and leads to spinal problems and brittle bones. But by doing regular exercises and by keeping yourself physically active you can prevent the bones from getting weaker. Through regular exercises you can also increase your physical stamina, improve your posture and get relief from joint pain. But you need to find exercises which are low impact and safe but at the same time effective in keeping the bones and muscles healthy.

Seek doctor's advice before you start following an exercise routine meant for osteoporosis. He may ask undergo a fitness test and a bone density test before he gives you the green signal.

Exercises for people with osteoporosis

There are three types of exercises which osteoporosis patients can follow:

Weight bearing aerobic activities

Strength training exercises

Flexibility exercises

Weight Bearing Aerobic Activities

This type of activities include the aerobic exercises which done while standing on the feet like climbing up the stairs, walking, gardening, working out on elliptical machines etc. This type of exercises offer a great workout for the legs, lower back and hips and also help to reduce mineral loss from bones. They also improve blood circulation in the body and help to keep the heart healthy.

Strength Training

Working out with resistance bands, weight machines and free weights will help you to strengthen your bones and muscles in your arms and spine. Through strength training you can keep your bones active and slow the process of mineral loss.

Flexibility Exercises

Through flexibility exercises you can increase the mobility of your joints and prevent stiffness and injury of muscles. When your body becomes flexible you will find it easy to sit and move in the right posture. But when your muscles and joints are stiff you tend to have a stooping posture.

Make your body flexible by doing stretches at end of every exercise routine. By doing stretches you can relax the muscles and joints and release the stress from your body.

EXERCISES TO BE AVOIDED BY OSTEOPOROSIS PATIENT:

High Impact Exercises

Avoid running, jogging and jumping. This type of exercises involves jerky and fast movements which can fracture your spinal cord and other fragile parts of the body. Since with age you will lose bone density you need to choose exercises which involves slow and steady movements.

Avoid Bending and Twisting Exercises

You should stay away from exercises which involves steps like bending forward to touch your toes, doing sit ups and twisting your waists. These exercises will put excess pressure on your spinal cord and may cause severe fracture. Also avoid other strenuous physical activities like tennis, yoga, bowling and golf.

People with osteoporosis have a high risk of getting a fracture, so they need to get an approval from their doctor before they start working out. The best would be to have a personal fitness trainer. He will test your physical condition and stamina and accordingly draw up a suitable exercise routine for you and can guide you properly during workouts.

Exercise is a very good way to improve a person's bone health. Any physical activity affects our bones, either increasing bone mass or changing bone structure.

Different types of exercise and sports affect different bone areas depending on what body part is used in the specific activity. Walking and running load the bones of the legs and lower back. On the other hand, swimming and ball games such as tennis, volleyball and baseball load the bones of the upper body. As a result of this exercises, bones are loaded eventually changing its structure. Bones also become thicker, stronger and less vulnerable to fracture and breaking. For children and younger people, a regular routine done or sports played will help them develop tougher bones and they will have a bone reserve when they become older.

The rule of the thumb in every exercise is that it should be more strenuous than one's daily activities. It is not enough that you do it regularly but also with more intensity, increased difficulty level and number of exercise. You shouldn't focus only on one type of exercise or sport but do a variety or combinations so that all bone areas are affected. For older people, being physically active or having an active lifestyle is necessary to prevent osteoporosis.

Here are some examples of exercises you can do to improve bone health:

In a supine position (lying on a mat), stretch yourself as long as possible for 5-10seconds. Then, put your arms behind your neck and bend the knees, lift your head for 5-10 times. Lastly, lift your hip while your arms remain stretched on the floor and legs are bent.

In a sitting position, stand up with arm support for 5-10 times. Then stand without any arm support for the same number of repetition.

BEFORE YOU START

Consult your doctor before starting any exercise program for osteoporosis. You might need some tests first, including:

Bone density measurement

Fitness assessment

In the meantime, think about what kind of activities you enjoy most. If you choose an exercise you enjoy, you're more likely to stick with it over time.

Choosing The Right Form Of Exercise

These types of activities are often recommended for people with osteoporosis:

Strength training exercises, especially those for the upper back

Weight-bearing aerobic activities

Flexibility exercises

Stability and balance exercises Because of the varying degrees of osteoporosis and the risk of fracture, you might be discouraged from doing certain exercises. Ask your doctor or physical therapist whether you're at risk of osteoporosis-related problems, and find out what exercises are appropriate for you.

STRENGTH TRAINING

Strength training includes the use of free weights, resistance bands or your own body weight to strengthen all major muscle groups, especially spinal muscles important for posture. Resistance training can also help maintain bone density.

If you use weight machines, take care not to twist your spine while performing exercises or adjusting the machines.

Resistance training should be tailored to your ability and tolerance, especially if you have pain. A physical therapist or personal trainer with experience working with people with osteoporosis can help you develop strength-training routines. Proper form and technique are crucial to prevent injury and get the most from your workout.

WEIGHT-BEARING AEROBIC ACTIVITIES

Weight-bearing aerobic activities involve doing aerobic exercise on your feet, with your bones supporting your weight. Examples include walking, dancing, low- impact aerobics, elliptical training machines, stair climbing and gardening. These types of exercise work directly on the bones in your legs, hips and lower spine to slow mineral loss. They also provide cardiovascular benefits, which boost heart and circulatory system health.

It's important that aerobic activities, as beneficial as they are for your overall health, are not the whole of your exercise program. It's also important to work on strength, flexibility and balance. Swimming and cycling have many benefits, but they don't provide the weight-bearing load your bones need to slow mineral loss. However, if you enjoy these activities, do them. Just be sure to also add weight-bearing activity as you're able.

FLEXIBILITY EXERCISES

Moving your joints through their full range of motion helps you keep your muscles working well. Stretches are best performed after your muscles are warmed up — at the end of your exercise session, for example, or after a 10-minute warm-up. They should be done gently and slowly, without bouncing.

Avoid stretches that flex your spine or cause you to bend at the waist. Ask your doctor which stretching exercises are best for you.

STABILITY AND BALANCE EXERCISES

Fall prevention is especially important for people with osteoporosis. Stability and balance exercises help your muscles work together in a way that keeps you more stable and less likely to fall. Simple exercises such as standing on one leg or movement-based exercises such as tai chi can improve your stability and balance.

Movements To Avoid

If you have osteoporosis, don't do the following types of exercises:

High-impact exercises. Activities such as jumping, running or jogging can lead to fractures in weakened bones. Avoid jerky, rapid movements in general.

Choose exercises with slow, controlled movements. If you're generally fit and strong despite having osteoporosis, however, you might be able to engage in somewhat higher-impact exercise than can someone who is frail.

Bending and twisting. Exercises in which you bend forward at the waist and twist your waist, such as touching your toes or doing sit-ups, can increase your risk of compression fractures in your spine if you have osteoporosis. Other activities that may re□uire you to bend or twist forcefully at the waist are golf, tennis, bowling and some yoga poses.

If you're not sure how healthy your bones are, talk to your doctor. Don't let fear of fractures keep you from having fun and being active.

Living with Osteoporosis: 8 Exercises to Strengthen Your Bones

While most types of exercise are good for you, not all types are good for healthy bones. For example, weight-bearing exercises can build healthy bone. These exercises involve challenging your muscle strength against gravity and putting pressure on your bones.

As a result, your bones will signal your body to produce added tissue to build stronger bones. Exercises such as walking or swimming may be beneficial to your lung and heart health but won't necessarily help you strengthen your bones.

Anyone with osteoporosis who's looking to increase their bone strength can benefit from the following eight exercises. These exercises are easy to do at home.

1. Foot Stomps

The goal for exercise to reduce osteoporosis is to challenge the key areas of your body that osteoporosis most commonly affects, such as your hips. One way to challenge your hip bones is through foot stomps. While standing, stomp your foot, imagining you are crushing an imaginary can underneath it.

Repeat four times on one foot, then repeat the exercise on the other foot.

Hold on to a railing or sturdy piece of furniture if you have difficulty maintaining your balance.

2. Bicep Curls

You can perform bicep curls with either dumbbells weighing between 1 to 5 pounds or a resistance band. They can be performed seated or standing, depending on what you're most comfortable with.

Take a dumbbell in each hand. Or step on a resistance band while holding an end in each hand.

Pull the bands or weights in toward your chest, watching the bicep muscles on the fronts of your upper arms contract.

Lower your arms to return to your starting position.

Repeat eight to 12 times. Rest and repeat for a second set, if possible.

3. Shoulder Lifts

You'll also need weights or a resistance band to perform shoulder lifts. You can do this exercise from either a standing or seated position. Take a dumbbell in each hand. Or step on a resistance band while holding an end in each hand.

Start with your arms down and hands at yoursides.

Slowly raise your arms out straight in front of you, but don't lock your elbow.

Lift to a comfortable height, but no higher than shoulder level.

Repeat eight to 12 times. Rest and repeat for a second set, if possible.

4. Hamstring Curls

Hamstring curls strengthen the muscles in the backs of your upper legs. You perform this exercise from a standing position. If necessary, place your hands on a piece of heavy furniture or other sturdy item to improve your balance.

Stand with your feet shoulder-width apart.

Slightly move back your left foot until only your toes are touching the floor.

Contract the muscles in the back of your left leg to lift your left heel toward your buttocks. Slowly control your left foot as you lower it back to its starting position.

Repeat the exercise between eight and 12 times.

Rest, and repeat the exercise on your right leg.

5. Hip Leg Lifts

This exercise strengthens the muscles around your hips as well as enhances your balance. Place your hands on a piece of heavy furniture or other sturdy item to improve your balance as needed.

Start with your feet hip-width apart. Shift your weight to your left foot.

Flex your right foot and keep your right leg straight as you lift it to the side, no more than 6 inches off the ground.

Lower your right leg.

Repeat the leg lift eight to 12 times. Return to your starting position and do another set using your left leg.

6. Squats

Squats can strengthen the front of your legs as well as your buttocks. You don't have to squat deeply for this exercise to be effective.

Start with your feet hip-width apart. Rest your hands lightly on a sturdy piece of

furniture or counter for balance.

Bend at your knees to slowly squat down. Keep your back straight and lean slightly forward, feeling your legs

working.

Squat only until your thighs are parallel to the ground.

Tighten your buttocks to return to a standing position.

Repeat this exercise eight to 12 times.

7. Ball Sit

This exercise can promote balance and strengthen your abdominal muscles. It should be performed with a large exercise ball. You should also have someone with you to act as a —spotter to help you maintain your balance.

Sit on the exercise ball with your feet flat on the floor.

Keep your back as straight as possible while you maintain your balance.

If you are able, hold your arms out at your sides, palms facing forward.

Hold the position as long as one minute, if possible. Stand and rest. Repeat the exercise up to two more times.

8. Standing on one leg

This exercise promotes greater balance. With a sturdy piece of furniture nearby if you need to grab onto something, stand on one foot for one minute, if possible.

Repeat the balance exercise on your other leg.

Importance of Weight-Bearing Exercises for Osteoporosis

Weight-bearing exercises help with the maintenance of strong bones because it triggers the production of hormones that stimulate bone production. Bone density is typically highest in younger

individuals, especially in those who move more and participate in sports and other types of physical activity. As you age your bones start to lose density, but you can slow this process with weight bearing exercises. Studies suggest that exercise helps to increase bone density by initiating pathways in the body that lead to bone production.

Chapter 12: Best Exercise For Osteoporosis

It's never too late to start a bone-healthy exercise program, even if you already have osteoporosis. You may worry that being active means you're more likely to fall and break a bone. But the opposite is true. A regular, properly designed exercise program may actually help prevent falls and fractures.

That's because exercise strengthens bones and muscles and improves balance, coordination, and flexibility. That's key for people with osteoporosis.

Check With Your Doctor

Before you start a new workout routine, check with your doctor and physical therapist. They can tell you what's safe for your stage of osteoporosis, your fitness level, and your general health.

There is no single exercise plan that's best for everyone with osteoporosis. The routine you choose should be unique to you and based on your:

Fracture risk

Muscle strength

Range of motion

Level of physical activity

Fitness

Gait

Balance

Your doctor also will consider any other health problems that have a bearing on your ability to exercise, such as obesity, high blood pressure, and heart disease. They may refer you to a specially trained physical therapist who can teach you exercises that focus on body mechanics and posture, balance, resistance weights, and other techniques.

Weight-Bearing Exercises for Osteoporosis

Don't let the name fool you -- these types of workouts aren't about pumping iron. They are exercises you do on your feet so that your bones and muscles have to work against gravity to keep you upright. Your bones react to the weight on them by building themselves up and getting stronger.

There are two types of weight-bearing exercise: high-impact and low-impact. High-impact includes workouts like:

Jogging

Jumping rope

Step aerobics

Tennis or other racquet sports

Yard work, like pushing a lawnmower or heavy gardening

Moderate impact exercises may include:

Climbing stairs

Dancing

Hiking

But be careful. If your osteoporosis is severe, high-impact weight-bearing exercises may not be safe for you.

Talk to your doctor about your workout routine. They may recommend that you focus on low-impact exercises that are less likely to cause fractures and still build up your bone density. These include:

Elliptical training machines

Low-impact aerobics

Stair-step machines

Walking (either outside or on a treadmill machine)

If you're new to exercise or haven't worked out for a while, you should aim to gradually increase the amount you do until you get to 30 minutes of weight-bearing exercise per day on most days of the week.

Strengthen Your Muscles

Working your muscles matters because it may help prevent fall-related fractures. Functional strength and balance training should be part of your routine.

These workouts can include basic moves such as standing and rising on your toes, lifting your own body weight with exercises like push-ups or squats, and using equipment such as:

Elastic exercise bands

Free weights

Weight machines

Add strength-training exercises to your workouts 2 to 3 days per week.

Non-Impact Exercises

These moves don't directly strengthen your bones. They can, though, improve your coordination and flexibility. That will lower the chance that you'll fall and break a bone. You can do these every day.

Balance exercises such as Tai Chi can strengthen your leg muscles and help you stay steadier on your feet. Posture exercises can help you work against the "sloping" shoulders that can happen with osteoporosis and lower your chances of spine fractures.

Routines such as yoga and Pilates can improve strength, balance, and flexibility in people with osteoporosis. But some of the moves you do in these programs including forward-bending exercises can make you more likely to get a fracture.

If you're interested in these workouts, talk with your doctor and ask your physical therapist to tell you the moves that are safe and those you should avoid.

Exercise can benefit almost everyone with osteoporosis. But remember it's only one part of a good treatment plan. Get plenty of calcium and vitamin D in your diet, stay at a healthy weight, and don't smoke or drink too much alcohol. You also may need osteoporosis medications to either build or maintain your bone density. Work with your doctor to figure out the best ways to stay healthy and strong.

When Too Much Exercise Can Be Bad for Bones

Some evidence shows that too much exercise can lead to bone problems, too. Intense training can cause hormone imbalances, which can lead to lower bone mass, called osteopenia. This can be a problem for some young female athletes. A balance of exercise and recovery is crucial to keeping osteoporosis at bay.

What Else You Can Do for Bone Health

Exercise can benefit almost everyone with osteoporosis. But remember it's only one part of a good treatment plan. Get plenty of calcium and vitamin D in your diet, stay at a healthy weight, and don't smoke or drink too much alcohol. You also may need osteoporosis medications to either build or maintain your bone density. Work with your doctor to figure out the best ways to stay healthy and strong.

Osteoporosis Exercise For Strong Bones

Staying active and exercising helps to stengthen muscles and improve overall bone health. There are two types of osteoporosis exercises that are important for building and maintaining bone density: weight- bearing and muscle-strengthening

exercises.

WEIGHT-BEARING EXERCISES

These exercises include activities that make you move against gravity while staying upright. Weight-bearing exercises can be high-impact or low- impact. High-impact weight-bearing exercises help build bones and keep them strong.

If you have broken a bone due to osteoporosis or are at risk of breaking a bone, you may need to avoid high-impact exercises.

If you're not sure, you should check with your healthcare provider.

Examples of high-impact weight-bearing exercises are:

Dancing

Doing high-impact aerobics

Hiking Jogging/running Jumping Rope Stair climbing Tennis

Low-impact weight-bearing exercises can also help keep bones strong and are a safe alternative if you cannot do high- impact exercises. Examples of low- impact weight-bearing exercises are:

Using elliptical training machines Doing low-impact aerobics

Using stair-step machines

Fast walking on a treadmill or outside

Muscle-Strengthening Exercises

These exercises include activities where you move your body, a weight or some other resistance against gravity. They are also known as resistance exercises and include:

Lifting weights

Using elastic exercise bands Using weight machines

Lifting your own body weight

Functional movements, such as standing and rising up on your toes

Exercise and Bone Health Osteoporosis is a common bone disease which makes your bones more fragile.

This increases the chance of you breaking a bone (also called a fracture), even with a minor bump or fall.

Osteoporosis may also cause you to lose height, and your posture to become stooped.

BALANCE EXERCISES

Improving your balance makes it less likely that you will fall. Balance, like everything else, takes practise to improve. Dancing and exercise to music classes can help improve your balance.

Tai Chi is another good way of improving your balance.

EXERCISES FOR GENERAL HEALTH

To mprove your general health, you need to be physically active to the point you

are slightly out of breath for about 30 minutes on most days. You don't have to do this all at once but can, for example, add up three ten minute activities. Start slowly and gradually build up. Start by setting aside 5 or 10 minutes, gradually increasing to 30 minutes of continuous activity. Physical activity not only includes exercise, but also daily activities like walking, climbing stairs, housework, gardening etc.

SWIMMING AND CYCLING

These exercises are non weight-bearing and therefore do not improve your bone density. However, they can improve your fitness and general health, so they are still good to do, but make sure you are doing some weight-bearing exercise too. What kind of exercise should I avoid?

Some exercises and activities put you at risk of injuring yourself, or at worst, breaking a bone. They include:

running, jogging, skipping, jumping and hopping

high impact aerobics

repeated forward bending (eg touching your toes)

fast twisting movements

any exercise that is likely to cause you to fall

Tips For Exercising

Always wear well-fitting footwear with cushioned soles or in-soles, such as trainers, when you are exercising.

Make sure the room is at a comfortable

temperature.

Always start with a gradual warm-up, followed by gentle stretches.

Always start slowly and gently. Build up gradually, working within your limits.

Pace yourself.

Keep breathing properly and don't hold your breath.

Although you may already have some discomfort, stop if the exercise increases or changes your pain in any way. If you begin to feel unwell during the exercise programme, do not continue. If this happens again, consult your GP.

If you become tired, instead of stopping, try slowing down.

Do the exercises in a controlled manner.

Find an activity that suits you. There is no point in forcing yourself to do something that you do not enjoy as it will be unlikely you will continue with it long term. Try out a few different ways of exercising to find out what you enjoy the most.

If you are exercising for the first time, you should see your GP first.

Home Exercise Programme

The exercises that follow are designed for you to do at home. It is important that you do them regularly (at least 3 times weekly) to improve then maintain, your posture, flexibility, strength and balance.

Before starting your exercises there are some important points to remember:

Make sure you are wearing well-fitting, supportive footwear.

Pace yourself, only do as many of the exercises as you feel comfortable with

Do the exercises slowly in a controlled manner.

Keep breathing properly and don't hold your breath during the exercise

If you begin to feel unwell during the exercise programme, do not continue. If this happens again consult your GP.

The exercises should not increase or change your pain in any way; you should be able to work within pain-free limits.

If this does occur, stop exercising. If this happens again consult your GP.

Chapter 13: Understanding Broken Bones

For our every day sports as humans, we rely at the electricity and flexibility of our bones and joints. Accidents, as an alternative, can motive these robust structures to turn out to be brittle, that could cause the scary occurrence of broken bones. We will discover the reasons, kinds, and ability effects of broken joints in this financial catastrophe, delving into their complex international.

The Dangerous Balance:

Our skeletal gadget, which offers mobility, safety, and guide, is an engineering surprise. Bones are extra than definitely mechanical structures; They are living tissues which might be constantly changing and adjusting to our desires. Nonetheless, under particular conditions, this touchy equilibrium can be disturbed, prompting cracks and broken joints.

What Causes Broken Bones?

Joint fractures may be attributable to a big variety of factors. Traumatic sports like falls, sports injuries, and automobile injuries can put too much strain at the bones, decreasing their resilience. Also, fantastic ailments like osteoporosis, growths, or ailments can debilitate bones, making them extra helpless to breaks regardless of insignificant effect.

Common Kinds of Broken Joints:

It is critical to understand the effects of the various kinds of broken joints for restoration and recovery. Breaks can pass from simple breaks to greater complicated breaks that encompass relocation, commutation, or the front of encompassing tissues. Each type calls for first rate treatment strategies custom-made to the singular's unique damage.

How it impacts the frame:

In addition to inflicting acute pain, a broken joint additionally makes it difficult for us to perform everyday activities. The diploma of impairment varies based totally truely at the fracture's severity and the joint affected. Restricted portability, increasing, swelling, and deformation are ordinary consequences, and whenever left untreated, complexities, as an example, nerve damage or debilitated blood route can emerge.

Looking for Clinical Consideration:

It is crucial to are seeking out set off clinical interest and recognize the signs and symptoms and signs of a broken joint for effective treatment. Inadequate restoration, lengthy-time period headaches, and extended ache can give up end result from delaying assessment and remedy. Through this element, we are capable of direct you on distinguishing whilst to look for proficient help and the manner to offer quick emergency treatment until clinical assistance is available.

Effect on intellectual health:

The mental and emotional toll of a damaged joint can not be overstated. Mental well-being can undergo due to handling pain, dependence on others, and frustration because of confined motion. It is critical for address the near home a part of recovery and foster methodologies to adapt to the issues that emerge in the course of the mending machine.

The basis for the following chapters, in which we will delve into powerful guides for recuperation and getting better from excessive pain, is an statistics of the fundamentals of broken joints. By gaining information approximately the motives, sorts, impacts, and the significance of searching out scientific hobby, we are capable of go away on an tour towards a fruitful healing and recapture our team spirit, portability, and private satisfaction.

Chapter 14: Immediate First Aid For Broken Joints

In a depend wide variety of seconds, an sudden disaster can bring about a tousled joint, inflicting large torment and distress. Having the abilities and information to provide instantaneous first aid need to make a large distinction in how an harm is going at the same time as it's so essential. In this bankruptcy, we will speak about the most critical steps to take at the same time as dealing with a damaged joint, together with the way to stabilize the damage and take away pain.

When confronted with a idea broken joint, it's miles vital to maintain quiet and focused. Keep in mind that appearing quick can assist save you further harm and offer the injured person with the an lousy lot-wished comfort. When administering immediately first aid, the subsequent have to be considered:

Evaluate What is going on:

Pause for a minute to assess the scene and assure your protection further to that of the harmed character. Remove any ability risks that might worsen the state of affairs, like sharp gadgets or volatile systems, if vital.

Speak up and reassure:

Engage with the injured individual and reassure them. Let them comprehend that they'll be now not by myself and that assistance is at the way. During this trying time, being able to speak brazenly can help reduce their anxiety and foster a greater upbeat outlook.

Put the joint out of motion:

The affected joint have to be immobilized to save you further damage. To stabilize the joint, lightly help the injured location collectively together with your palms or, if to be had, use improvised splints. Be cautious not to vicinity an excessive amount of stress on the joint or circulate it too much because of the truth doing so have to make the harm worse.

Reduce Swelling and Bleeding:

Use a easy fabric or sterile dressing to use slight stress to prevent seen bleeding. Lifting the harmed appendage, if feasible, can likewise help with lessening growing. However, avoid excessive joint manipulation.

Use cold compression:

To lighten torment and reduce enlarging, using a virulent disease p.C. Or ice percent to the harmed place can be beneficial. Wrap the ice % in a cloth or towel and put it delicately at the joint for spherical 15 to 20 minutes , with time within the middle among.

Assist with Pain Relief:

Assuming the harmed individual is encountering important torment, you may manage over-the-counter ache killers, following the counseled length. Nonetheless, it's miles important to signify a hospital therapy talented preceding to giving any prescription, specially at the off risk that the man or woman has hidden ailments or takes one-of-a-type meds.

Look for Clinical Consideration:

Although right away first useful aid measures are important, they have to no longer take the location of expert clinical attention. As quick as possible, touch emergency services or transport the injured individual to the closest sanatorium. Further assessment of the harm, diagnostic tests, and the great direction of treatment for pinnacle-rated recuperation can be determined thru clinical professionals.

Keep in thoughts that the steps on this bankruptcy are supposed to help proper away till expert clinical help arrives. A broken joint calls for widespread medical remedy, rehabilitation, and prolonged-time period care, all of so one may be cited in next chapters. You can play a important feature in making sure the properly-being and comfort of a person with a damaged joint with the resource of studying the manner to offer at once first useful resource.

Chapter 15: Diagnosing And Assessing The Severity Of Broken Joints

When confronted with a suspicion of a damaged joint, it is essential to determine the quantity of the harm and advantage an accurate prognosis. This chapter affords a foundation for making suitable remedy choices by way of focusing at the crucial steps involved in diagnosing and assessing the amount of a broken joint. By know-how the analytic cycle, human beings and hospital treatment specialists can effectively oversee damaged joints and begin the manner to restoration.

Identifying Symptoms:

Perceiving the signs and symptoms and side effects of a tousled joint is the most vital section in the symptomatic cycle. Intense pain, swelling, deformity, bruising, trouble transferring the joint, and a vital change in look are all not unusual symptoms. It is vital to maintain in mind that some fractures may not display up as apparent deformities, necessitating a whole exam to confirm the prognosis.

Examining the frame:

After thinking a messed up joint, a clinic treatment gifted will carry out a whole actual evaluation. They will cautiously survey the harmed vicinity, trying to find signs of delicacy, precariousness, crepitus (crushing or breaking sensations), or odd improvement. Comparing the injured joint to the wholesome joint can help find out versions and abnormalities.

Exams for photos:

To confirm the presence of a crack and decide its vicinity and seriousness, it are frequently applied to photograph tests. The most commonplace imaging approach for diagnosing damaged joints is X-rays. They provide centered pictures of the bones, making it feasible for scientific experts to end up aware about fractures, examine alignment, and study any complications that can be associated with them, along side joint dislocation or bone displacement.

Now and yet again, greater imaging modalities is probably used, contingent upon the person and intricacy of the harm. Ultrasound, computed tomography (CT), and magnetic resonance imaging (MRI) are examples of these. These tests help determine whether or not or not or not a ligament or tendon has been broken through imparting a higher have a study the smooth tissues that surround the joint.

Expertise Consultation:

A consultation with an orthopedic expert can be required for immoderate or complicated fractures. These experts have ability in overseeing damaged joints and may supply crucial testimonies into the most becoming remedy options. In order to absolutely recognize the harm and its consequences, they will advocate more tests or opinions.

Assessing the severity and available treatments:

The severity of the fracture is probably determined thru manner of healthcare specialists based totally mostly on the analysis and evaluation of the broken joint. Fractures are damaged down into classes based totally completely totally on their complexity, area, displacement, and involvement of the tissues that surround them. From non-surgical strategies like casting or splinting to surgical interventions like open reduce charge and internal fixation or outside fixation, this kind aids in making treatment alternatives.

Ideas for Recovering and Healing:

Healthcare specialists will recollect a variety of things that can have an effect on recovery and recovery further to figuring out the severity of the broken joint. The man or woman's age, way of lifestyles, and everyday health are all examples of those elements. Healthcare professionals can tailor the treatment plan and provide suitable steering for rehabilitation and lengthy-term recovery with this knowledge.

In this detail, we have investigated the pivotal advances engaged with diagnosing and surveying the seriousness of broken joints. By perceiving thing results, directing real checks, using imaging checks, and speakme with hassle rely professionals, medical services experts can decide knowledgeable alternatives close to therapy and supply human beings the maximum obvious possibility for a fruitful restoration. In the chapters that come after this one, we're able to take a deeper have a look at useful manuals and strategies for repairing broken joints, controlling pain, and regaining mobility.

Chapter 16: Treating Broken Joints
Medical Interventions And Procedures

For most exciting restoration and healing from a damaged joint, prompt and appropriate medical treatment is essential. The severa remedy options for broken joints, from non-surgical techniques to surgical strategies, are examined in Chapter 4. By data the ones intercessions, people and clinical services specialists can go with knowledgeable picks regarding the cheapest technique for every specific case.

Alternative Therapies:

Immobilization: For specific varieties of cracks, immobilization is the critical remedy technique. Casts, splints, or braces are used to hold the broken joint solid and permit the bones to align and heal on their very personal. Regular have a look at-up visits are often made after immobilization to assess improvement and make any crucial modifications.

Traction: Traction can be carried out in greater complex fractures or whilst alignment wants to be restored. Footing includes the delicate pulling force finished to the messed up joint, regularly using loads and pulleys. This method aids in realigning the bones and alleviates pressure at the tissues round them, thereby facilitating restoration.

Reduced Closed: To realign displaced fractures, a closed discount system is used in location of surgical remedy. The bones are carefully repositioned with the beneficial aid of healthcare professionals via manual manipulation. To lessen pain and ache, this is commonly completed beneath community or present day day anesthesia.

Surgical Procedures:

Open Decrease and Inward Obsession (ORIF): Surgical intervention may be required if the fracture is excessive, volatile, or followed through tremendous displacement. In ORIF, an incision is made close to the damaged joint, the bones are realigned, and screws, plates, or rods are used to preserve them in region. This gives stability and empowers suitable improving.

Fixation from Outside: When inner fixation isn't possible or suitable, an opportunity surgical approach is used. This consists of setting pins or wires into the bone above and beneath the fracture. These pins or wires are then linked to a frame that is outside the frame. The damaged joint can heal properly due to the fact the body maintains it stable.

Replacement joints: Joint substitute surgical treatment may be considered if the broken joint is significantly broken or cannot be repaired. This includes getting rid of the harmed joint and supplanting it with a fake joint, like an embed or prosthesis. The reason of joint replacement surgical procedure is to restore mobility, lessen ache, and repair characteristic.

Procedures with Little to No Incisions: Certain fractures can now be treated with minimally invasive techniques manner to improvements in clinical era. To restore the broken joint, those techniques use small incisions, specialized gadgets, and guided imaging. Negligibly obvious techniques regularly result in an entire lot much less tissue damage, faster recuperation, and diminished scarring.

Considerations Following Treatment:

Proper submit-treatment care is essential for promoting recovery and maximizing restoration following any remedy for a broken joint. Typically, this includes a complete rehabilitation plan tailor-made to the character's particular requirements. Physical treatment, bodily video games to increase power and range of motion, ache control techniques, and education on regularly returning to ordinary sports can also all be part of rehabilitation.

Chapter 17: Non-Surgical Approaches To Healing Broken Joints

Non-surgical treatments for broken joints are clearly as critical as scientific interventions and surgical strategies. These non-surgical treatments, which may be used on my own or at the factor of different interventions, are the point of interest of Chapter five. Individuals can advantage insight into possibility options for correctly treating pain and recovery broken joints via reading those strategies.

Physical remedy and rehabilitation:

Restoration and energetic recuperation are vital additives of non-careful remedy for broken joints. The goals of those remedies are to strengthen the encircling muscle corporations and tissues, repair mobility, and repair characteristic. Physical therapists create individualized workout regimens that target specific muscle corporations and joint movements. They lead human beings through a whole lot of bodily sports activities, stretches, and strategies to regain energy, flexibility, and range of motion. In addition, modalities like warmness or cold remedy, ultrasound, and electrical stimulation are carried out in rehabilitation to speed up healing and decrease ache.

Techniques for Bearing Weight and Reducing Stress:

Weight-bearing and stress-lessening techniques can be helpful in some unspecified time in the future of the mending tool of a messed up joint. Healthcare experts can also recommend partial weight-bearing or non-weight-bearing activities to guard the joint and encourage bone restoration, counting on the severity and place of the fracture. To lessen joint strain whilst transferring, assistive devices like crutches, walkers, or canes may be used. These strategies paintings with a slow getting decrease again to everyday carrying sports, forestalling extra harm and advancing a fruitful recuperation.

Sustenance and Supplementation:

Legitimate sustenance assumes a notable element in the mending system of damaged joints. An even eating recurring plentiful in crucial dietary dietary supplements, together with vitamins (mainly diet plan D and C), minerals (like calcium and magnesium), and protein, upholds bone nicely being and allows in tissue restoration. For the motive of making sure an right enough deliver of essential nutrients and assisting the restoration and strengthening of bones and joints, clinical specialists might also furthermore in some instances advocate specific nutritional dietary supplements.

Torment The executives Techniques:

During the healing segment, powerful pain manipulate is important. Non-cautious strategies to address torment the board for damaged joints encompass the usage of non-steroidal mitigating capsules (NSAIDs) to decrease pain and irritation. These prescriptions can be recommended or to be had with out a prescription, yet it's miles critical to observe the suggested size and speak with a hospital therapy gifted if important. Additionally, topical analgesics, acupuncture, and exclusive alternative strategies of ache manage like transcutaneous electric powered nerve stimulation (TENS) may also additionally provide a few individuals with comfort.

Assistive Gadgets and Orthotics:

Assistive devices and orthotics can provide assist and stability at some level in the getting better device of broken joints. Braces, splints, or specialised orthotic devices can be recommended to immobilize and defend the injured area, depending on the affected joint. These devices help with decreasing struggling, forestall in addition harm, and enhance mending with the resource of the use of presenting help and stability to the joint.

Lifestyle changes:

To useful resource inside the healing of a damaged joint, positive way of lifestyles changes can be required inside the direction of the healing section. Maintaining a healthy weight to reduce joint pressure, making sure right body mechanics and ergonomics, running in the path of rest techniques to lessen muscle tension, and keeping off sports activities that positioned an excessive amount of pressure at the joint are all examples of those adjustments.

Individuals can actively participate in their recuperation, beautify recovery, and beautify their tremendous exquisite of lifestyles with the resource of incorporating those non-surgical treatments into the remedy plan for a damaged joint. It is possible to get the most out of those non-surgical remedies via working cautiously with medical specialists and following the commands.

Chapter 18: Rehabilitation And Physical Therapy For Broken Joints

To heal damaged joints, surgical strategies are required while non-surgical strategies are insufficient or beside the point. The severa surgical techniques used to deal with intense fractures and make sure a quick recovery are said good sized in Chapter 6. Individuals and healthcare specialists alike can benefit from an expertise of these techniques while considering surgical options for treating damaged joints.

Open Decrease and Inward Obsession (ORIF):

For the remedy of damaged joints with huge displacement, instability, or complex fractures, ORIF is a commonplace surgical remedy. An incision is made near the broken joint just so the clinical medical doctor can get to the damaged bones proper away. Internal fixation devices like screws, plates, rods, or wires are used to stabilize the joint after the bones are cautiously realigned. While the broken joint heals, the fixation devices provide help and stability.

Fixation from Outside:

Outside obsession is a careful device applied even as indoors obsession isn't possible or low-cost for the tousled joint. It includes the situation of pins or wires into the bone above and under the crack internet web web page. The broken joint is stabilized and aligned through using the ones pins or wires which can be related to an out of doors body outdoor the body. The outer fixator considers adjustments relying on the state of affairs during the getting higher gadget.

Replacement joints:

Joint possibility surgical operation can be encouraged if the damaged joint is seriously damaged or cannot be repaired. Joint substitution is composed of having rid of the harmed joint surfaces and supplanting them with counterfeit joint elements. These additives, called inserts or prostheses, are intended to duplicate the functionality and development of the everyday joint. The purpose of joint substitute surgery is to get joints strolling another time, get rid of pain, and be more mobile. Hip, knee, and shoulder replacements are most of the maximum common styles of joint replacements.

Osteotomy:

Osteotomy is a surgical remedy that includes the reshaping or repositioning of troubles that stays to be labored out affiliation and simplicity weight on the wrecked joint. When malalignment persists irrespective of particular treatments or for tremendous types of fractures, it is probably some thing to recall. By changing the bone shape surrounding the joint, osteotomy can assist in restoring joint stability, enhancing characteristic, and lowering ache.

Arthroscopy:

A minimally invasive surgery referred to as arthroscopy is used to diagnose and cope with quite a few joint conditions, at the side of a few types of fractures. Through tiny incisions, an arthroscope, a small, flexible tool, is inserted into the joint. The fashionable practitioner can use the arthroscope to appearance the systems of the joints and make the critical upkeep, which include realigning fractured bones, repairing torn ligaments, or getting rid of loose fragments. When in contrast to standard open surgical procedures, arthroscopic techniques generally have shorter recovery instances, lots less scarring, and much less tissue harm.

Care and Rehabilitation After Surgery:

For a success recovery from broken joint surgical treatment, proper submit-operative care and rehabilitation are vital. This regularly necessitates a multidisciplinary method that contains bodily treatment, rehabilitation sports, and ache management.